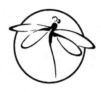

PRAISE FOR *THE TRANSFORMATION BOOK*

"Justin and Janell are authorities in their field. This is a must-read for anyone interested in making significant and impactful changes in their health and their life."

Dr. Jeffrey D. Algajer, D.C.
Owner, Discover Chiropractic Life Center

"With The Transformation Book, *Justin and Janell have provided you with the guide to the transformation you've been looking for. The Trans-*formation Book *delivers exactly what you need to understand to finally look and feel the way you want. And the best part is that it's practical, useful, and beneficial no matter how significant the transformation you want to make or what you've tried before."*

Pat Rigsby
Father, husband, entrepreneur, coach, and author

"The Transformation Book *is a must-read if you're finally ready to say 'Yes!' to you. Justin and Janell are leaders when it comes to the knowledge, experience, and passion they have in the areas of mind-set, fitness, and nutrition. This one book will single handedly change your life . . . when you let it."*

Jennifer Grant
Speaker, author, and coach

"If you're looking for another simplistic book, program, video, product, or gimmick, this is not for you. However, if you want to find the most successful strategies at achieving a true transformation, this is for you.

Justin and Janell aren't in the business of providing a mediocre experience and treating everyone with the same approach. They understand that in order to achieve true transformations, a program needs to be customized to the person striving for improvement. A one-size-fits-all approach just doesn't work.

A true transformation doesn't come from just eating better and getting your butt off the couch and going to the gym. Most people will bump up the exercise and start eating less when trying to lose weight, but what happens when you stall? Do you work out more and eat less? This approach can only work for so long. You simply can't keep cutting calories and increasing the intensity and volume of your training sessions.

The Transformation Book *helps elaborate on four distinct areas necessary for success. Not only does this book help you understand those four areas but it helps you learn how to customize to fit you and your individual needs. If you want to truly transform and develop the habits needed to be happy and healthy, you'll need to focus on mind-set, nutrition, exercise, and other lifestyle factors.* The Transformation Book *covers this and more, so if you're looking for a transformation, look no further. The title of the book says it all."*

Steve Long & Jared Woolever
Co-owners, Smart Group Training

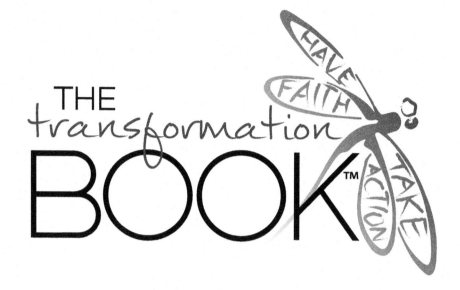

FOREWORD BY DR. BENJAMIN BAECHLER, MD

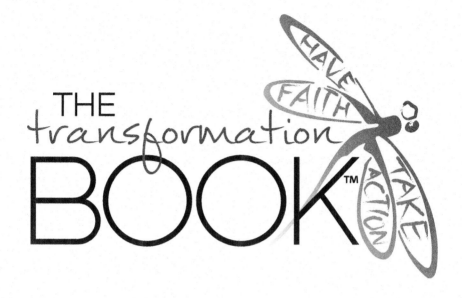

THE *transformation* BOOK™

A Proven 4-Part Plan to
Help You Lose Weight, Feel Great, and
Become the BEST Version of YOU!

JUSTIN YULE, BS, CPT, MTE, FMSC
JANELL YULE, BS, FDN-P, CPT

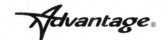

Published by Advantage, Charleston, South Carolina.
Member of Advantage Media Group.

ADVANTAGE is a registered trademark, and the Advantage colophon is a trademark of Advantage Media Group, Inc.

Printed in the United States of America.

ISBN: 978-1-59932-840-9
LCCN: 2016963036

Cover design by Katie Biondo.

This publication is designed to provide accurate and authoritative information in regard to the subject matter covered. It is sold with the understanding that the publisher is not engaged in rendering legal, accounting, or other professional services. If legal advice or other expert assistance is required, the services of a competent professional person should be sought.

Advantage Media Group is proud to be a part of the Tree Neutral® program. Tree Neutral offsets the number of trees consumed in the production and printing of this book by taking proactive steps such as planting trees in direct proportion to the number of trees used to print books. To learn more about Tree Neutral, please visit **www.treeneutral.com.**

Advantage Media Group is a publisher of business, self-improvement, and professional development books. We help entrepreneurs, business leaders, and professionals share their Stories, Passion, and Knowledge to help others Learn & Grow. Do you have a manuscript or book idea that you would like us to consider for publishing? Please visit **advantagefamily.com** or call **1.866.775.1696.**

To my father:

Thank you for introducing me to the gym
and being a role model for hard work and dedication.

To my mother:

Your compassion and support meant all the difference
as I pursued my passion and found my way through life.

—Justin

To my father:

I inherited your best qualities: your ability to
connect with people and your love of food.

To my mother:

You are my best friend! Much of my own health journey has been inspired by you;
know that what you are going through is helping others. I get my ability to cook from
you; thank you for encouraging me in the kitchen at such a young age.

—Janell

To the Members of The Transformation Club and our clients worldwide:
You are our inspiration as we strive every day to discover even better ways to educate,
motivate, and inspire you to become the BEST version of YOU.

—Justin & Janell

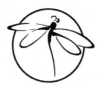

table of contents

Why We Chose a Dragonfly for Our Logo xi

Foreword xiii

Introduction 1

How to Get the Most out of This Book 15

Part 1: The Mind-Set Program 19

Chapter 1: It's All in Your Head 21

Chapter 2: What Do YOU Think? 25

Chapter 3: Thoughts & Things 33

Part 2: The Nutrition Program 43

Chapter 4: All Calories Are Not Created Equal . . . 45

Chapter 5: Hormones & Weight Loss 53

Chapter 6: Inflammation—Fighting the
Fire Within 61

Chapter 7: Just Eat Real Food 89

Chapter 8: Building a Solid
Nutrition Foundation 101

Chapter 9: The Truth about Carbohydrates 115

Chapter 10: Understanding Sugar 123

Chapter 11: Fat Is Your Friend 137

Chapter 12: Liquids 151

Chapter 13: Nutrition on the Go 157

Part 3: The Training Program **167**

Chapter 14: Stop Exercising If You Want
Long-Term Results. 169

Chapter 15: Resistance Training 183

Chapter 16: Cardio Training 197

Chapter 17: Setting Up Your Training Schedule. . . 209

Chapter 18: A Few Words about Warming Up. . . . 213

Chapter 19: How to Choose the Best
Exercises for You 221

Chapter 20: Your Transformation
Workout Program 229

Part 4: The Lifestyle Program **237**

Chapter 21: The Many Faces of Stress. 239

Chapter 22: Your Self-Care Toolbox. 251

Chapter 23: Mindful Eating 259

Chapter 24: An Attitude of Gratitude 267

Chapter 25: Managing Your Minimums 273

Chapter 26: Progress, Not Perfection 277

Chapter 27: Life beyond the Book 285

Afterword: It's *Not* about the Weight Loss **289**

How to Get Started **293**

Resources **295**

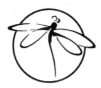

why we chose a dragonfly for our logo

The dragonfly, much like a butterfly, symbolizes change. In reality, we could have chosen a butterfly but felt that was a little too cliché and didn't fully represent what *The Transformation Club* (and now *The Transformation Book*) is about.

The dragonfly symbolizes change in the perspective of self-realization. This kind of change is much deeper than just a physical change.

You will experience powerful and positive, life-changing, mental and emotional changes, as well as a dramatic physical (better body) change as a Member of *The Transformation Club* and a reader of *The Transformation Book*.

The traditional association of dragonflies with water also gives rise to this deeper meaning.

The dragonfly's scurrying flight across water represents an act of going *beyond* what's on the surface and looking into the deeper implications and aspects of life.

You will find that implementing the techniques in *The Transformation Book* and being part of *The Transformation Club* will do so much more than just improve the way you look, feel, and perform.

You will see yourself in a completely different (better) light, which then shines on the lives of your family, friends, and coworkers.

The dragonfly's agile flight and its ability to move in all six directions exude a sense of power and poise.

For you, this translates into your ability to move like a kid again and get back to some of the fun activities you enjoyed in your youth before the aches and pains set in. Our Members who have kids and grandkids love that they can keep up with (and sometimes outperform) them.

The dragonfly exhibits iridescence both on its wings and its body. Iridescence is the property of an object to show itself in different colors depending on the angle and polarization of light falling on it. This property is seen and believed as the end of one's self-created illusions and a clear vision into the realities of life. The magical property of iridescence is also associated with the discovery of one's own abilities by unmasking the real self and removing the doubts one casts on his/her own sense of identity.

Deep stuff, we know.

For you, it means self-discovery and removal of inhibitions, a critical step in becoming *the BEST version of YOU!*

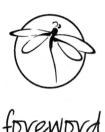

foreword

Life is a journey of transformation. In fact, we all are continually responding and changing as it relates to the world around us. Our experiences and individual actions shape our lives. More importantly, they shape and transform who we become.

But there is a secret…transformation occurs with or without our active involvement. The question is, "If we do not actively engage in the direction of our transformation, who do we become?" If we choose to be passive and allow ourselves to be victims of circumstance, our change will likely be one of regret and disappointment. Without active and positive engagement, we will never reach our potential. Unfortunately, many people never take or complete the steps necessary to move their lives forward with a sense of intentional direction and positive purpose. That is where *The Transformation Book*, written by Justin and Janell Yule, can make all the difference. It is a game changer for taking action.

I have known Justin and Janell for years. Their personal commitment to helping others bring out "the best version" of themselves is inspiring. Experts in physical and nutritional wellness, they have applied knowledge and cutting-edge techniques to help people achieve dramatic results. Yet, the best attribute of this dynamic team is their ability to serve as wellness coaches who provide not only the education but the motivation to help inspire others to achieve their goals. Driving them is the belief that we all are here to bring out the best in each other with our God-given talents.

The Transformation Book is an owner's manual for real results. The first section of the book strategically focuses on the mental mind-set needed for positive change. If one only read and applied this part of the book, that in itself would result in life-changing skills gained. Filled with concepts and content that creatively inspires the reader to reframe their mind-set, it is the basis for positively positioning one with newfound tools and enthusiasm. Following this, Justin and Janell provide an enjoyable journey through nutrition, physical training, and overall lifestyle choices, which gives the reader step-by-step instruction to accomplish their set goals. At the same time, Justin and Janell continually reinforce their own goals for the reader: to become the best version of themselves, to be happy, healthy, and fit.

One of the best parts of *The Transformation Book* is its emphasis on real world examples and easy-to-follow schedules for both food and fitness choices. In a world of incredibly confusing nutritional information, this guide helps the reader understand the impact of their dietary selections. Explaining how certain foods and their timing act in the body, the reader gains a new appreciation and reason to make different dietary choices. The key is helping the reader make their dietary, fitness, and lifestyle choices from a position of knowledge and strength. Justin and Janell do just that. With their colorful writing and heart-to-heart approach in conversation, one cannot help but feel as if Justin and Janell are enthusiastically standing close, saying, "You can do it!"

With thousands of lives positively changed by the knowledge and techniques outlined in this writing, *The Transformation Book* contains a "user-friendly" approach to get real results for real people (with real lives and jobs). If you are someone seeking to take a positive step forward in your life, simply read the first few pages of this book. You will be convinced of its value and won't be able to put it down!

I give *The Transformation Book* my highest recommendation and congratulate Justin and Janell on an outstanding resource for those seeking to transform their own lives.

With warmest wishes for well-being,
Benjamin J. Baechler, MD

introduction

If you're anything like us, this is *not* your first time reading a weight loss, fitness, diet, or exercise book. Combined, we've read hundreds.

So why is this book any different and why should you read it cover to cover?

Perhaps the most compelling reason is because, in truth, we're just like you—real people with busy lives who want a realistic program that provides real results.

Allow us to introduce ourselves . . .

JANELL YULE

BS, Health Promotion and Wellness, Psychology Minor
Functional Diagnostic Nutrition Practitioner

My relationship with food has been rocky, to say the least. I absolutely *love* food, but I once had the belief that food didn't love me.

I have struggled with my weight for as long as I can remember. I have *never* been the person who could "eat whatever they want." Growing up, I never looked the way I thought I should. Even though I was active in sports from fifth grade through high school, I never felt like I looked like an athlete. I remember middle school and the first couple years of high school being the worst. I hated shopping for clothes, and I just didn't feel comfortable in my own skin.

Food was my enemy because it made me overweight—at least, that was my thinking back then. I even went through a period in high school when I had very disordered eating habits. Looking back, it was much worse than I ever acknowledged to myself or to anyone else. I would avoid going to the cafeteria for lunch so I could avoid eating. When I did eat, I would pick at my food so it looked like I was eating, but really I wasn't. I would eat as little as possible for a few days, maybe a week, and then say, "Screw it!" and go on a binge. That cycle repeated over and over.

At the time, I had little idea what I was doing to my body. I just wanted to be thinner because my belief was if I was thinner I would be happier, more people would like me, I would have a boyfriend, and my popularity would increase. I put all of my self-worth into what my body looked like. If I was thin, I believed, then I was worthy of love, affection, and all of the things I desired in my life.

To be honest, I don't remember what snapped me out of this horrible cycle. All I know is that I was fortunate enough to know that starving myself was not the answer.

However, I still thought I needed to "restrict" what I ate and follow a low-fat diet. I followed the old *exercise more, eat less* approach. The problem with this approach was that I couldn't do it for more than a few days at time, maybe a few weeks if I really pushed myself to the edge.

RESTRICT › BINGE › FEEL BAD
ABOUT MYSELF › REPEAT

I thought there was something wrong with me because I couldn't stick to my diet. *I must be weak*, I thought. *I have no willpower.*

This behavior continued through college, except instead of starving myself I would exercise myself into the ground with endless hours of long, boring cardio workouts. That was strike two against my metabolism and hormones—which I know now are the keys to achieving and maintaining a healthy weight. By the way, all those hours of cardio coupled with my college shenanigans netted me about a *thirty-pound weight gain*! So much for that approach.

Strike three came after college. I focused on counting calories. Like many, I thought of weight loss as a simple mathematical formula: calories in vs. calories out. Besides being a poor approach in and of itself, my food choices were terrible. While I met my calorie or "points" requirements, I was literally poisoning my body with Frankenfoods (food-like substances) like Jimmy Dean breakfast sandwiches, Smart Ones, Subway, and my number-one nemesis for so many years: Diet Coke.

At this point, the side effects of my "diet" were much worse because I was working a stressful full-time job—sleeping until noon was no longer an option. I was exhausted all the time. I was moody and depressed, and my emotions were out of control. I also started to suffer from digestive issues, and my sleep patterns were a mess.

I tried to get a grip on things by going to my doctor for advice. With a shrug of the shoulders, she said, *"That's just how it is."*

Needless to say, I got the heck out of there and started looking beyond Western medicine and what I had been taught in traditional nutrition textbooks.

That's when my journey toward a whole food, supportive nutrition plan and lifestyle began. I began to dig into information on gluten, hormones, metabolism, stress, digestion, supplementation, sleep, and more.

The first big change I made to my diet was getting rid of Diet Coke, which was *not* easy! I did survive, though, and now I wouldn't touch it with a ten-foot pole.

Next, I started to pay attention to gluten. It took me about two years to get it completely out of my diet. The difference in how I feel now that I no longer eat gluten is truly amazing. The biggest change I noticed was in my emotions—I no longer have a tendency toward depression. I was depressed for many years and never made the connection that the food I was consuming was contributing to it.

From there, I began to question everything that I had known to be "healthy." I decided that if what I was doing wasn't working, then I needed to do something else. Einstein said, "The definition of insanity is doing the same thing over and over again and expecting a different result."

My focus switched to the quality of food that I ate instead of the quantity. I chose high-quality grass-fed beef and wild salmon over conventional meat and frozen fish. I made sure that the basis of my meals was protein and vegetables. This was a big deal because as a child I was one of the pickiest eaters ever! I would eat carrots and sometimes broccoli; that was the extent of my vegetable intake. After learning how beneficial vegetables were to my health and ability to lose weight, I stepped out of my comfort zone and tried new vegetables, as well as ways to prepare them. *Who would have thought veggies could be so good?*

As I was discovering the answers, I decided that I wanted to be a resource for others that were not getting the help they needed from conventional Western medicine. This is when I sought out my certification to become a Functional Diagnostic Nutrition Practitioner.

> "FDN is an emerging field and growing body of work that bridges the gap between clinical nutrition and functional medicine. It is a type of detective work that seeks to identify and correct the underlying causes and conditions that lead to an individual's main health complaints. FDN is not diagnosing or treating any disease nor practicing medicine."
>
> —Reed Davis, founder of Functional Diagnostic Nutrition

By eating *real* food, getting to bed on time, managing stress, and working out properly, I started seeing the results I've always wanted.

My journey involved several three- to six-week detoxes, where I completely eliminated foods that cause inflammation as well as foods that were triggers for me, such as baked goods. These "resets" taught me about the foods that worked for my body, how I was using food in my life, and my relationship to certain foods. The information that I gained from eliminating inflammatory foods, and then strategically reintroducing some of them, was invaluable.

I truly believe that for anyone to build their own supportive nutrition plan, they must take a period of time dedicated to elimination and then go through a reintroduction period. It is the only way for you to know what foods are working for you and which ones are not. It is not until you get certain foods completely out of your diet that you can identify how they are affecting your health and your weight.

Eating a real whole food diet void of processed foods has helped me achieve and maintain a healthy weight, plus it has provided me with *food freedom.*

Now when I choose to eat something I would not normally eat, such as ice cream, I can have a small amount and then move on. I am not haunted by the unfinished pint of ice cream in the freezer. I am able to make conscious choices about what goes in my body, and I have a level of awareness around food that was never present before.

Through many years of practice, I can identify the difference between physical hunger and psychological or emotional hunger. I can pause and ask myself, *What are you truly hungry for right now?* Often times, it is *not* food—instead I find that I am tired, need connection, or am feeling overwhelmed and/or stressed and think that food will allow me to feel better. And it will in the short term, which is why so many people reach for it. In today's fast-paced, stress-filled world, food has become how we deal with our emotions and comfort ourselves, instead of a way to nourish our bodies.

I no longer view food as the enemy, because I know the right types of foods to eat. I provide my body with nutrient-dense food so that I can feel and perform at my best. I still enjoy eating and love to cook, but the types of food I cook are different.

Instead of using exercise as a way to compensate for my unhealthy eating habits and focusing on working out to attain the "perfect" body, I move my body in ways that feel good to me physically, mentally, and emotionally. I no longer obsess about how many calories I am able to burn in a workout. I work out because I am blessed with a capable body that is able to move. My focus has shifted to what my body *can do*, rather than what my body *looks like*.

I no longer take an all-or-nothing approach to nutrition and fitness. In the past, if I didn't have at least one hour to dedicate to my workout, then forget it, it's not worth doing just part of it. As I write that, it sounds absolutely absurd but I don't think I am alone in this. How many times have you said, "I only have ten or twenty minutes to work out, so what's the point?"

Or taking the all-or-nothing approach to nutrition: "I already messed up today so I might as well eat what I want the rest of the day!" I would bet that you have had a similar conversation with yourself many times. The most common being, "I'll start on Monday!"

Through nutrition, supplementation, consistent exercise, and yoga, my cravings, digestive health, sleep, hormone balance, moods, and energy have all improved.

Changing what/how/when I eat and working out on a consistent basis hasn't always been easy and effortless, but it has been worth it!

I now eat and move in a way that I can do for the rest of my life. Eating a diet based around whole nutrient-dense foods and working out consistently is no longer something I *have* to do but rather something I *choose* to do because I love and respect myself.

I am grateful for the path that led me here, even the tough parts—they're what taught me the most. I am grateful for the knowledge and awareness I have gained. Living a healthy lifestyle is a journey, not a destination. I am still on my journey; I still don't have certain things mastered and I likely never will. Instead, I practice *progress not perfection* and strive to be the *best* version of myself every day!

Most importantly, I know that I am worth the time, energy, and money that go into eating a real, whole food supportive nutrition plan, working out consistently, self-care, and loving myself.

YOU are worth it, too!

JUSTIN YULE

BS, Physical Education, Concentration in Adult Fitness
Certified Personal Trainer

I originally got into fitness way back in 1988 as a "stocky" thirteen-year-old kid who just wanted to feel comfortable in his own skin. I hated being embarrassed to take my shirt off in the locker room or at the public pool. Being called "meatloaf" in eighth grade didn't help much either.

Now, I don't want to paint a picture that I was some morbidly obese kid with no life who locked himself in his bedroom all day. I was an active kid—pretty athletic, in fact—and was pretty popular with the ladies. But the truth was that **I was extremely self-conscious because of the way I looked.** Right or wrong, my self-image was terrible.

One day my dad invited me to go with him to his gym, the All American. It was your classic iron-pumping, weight-banging, meathead gym of the 1980s. It was awesome!

He introduced me around and, to my surprise, the guys were really welcoming. The owner even helped me develop my first training program. It was so cool! Being welcomed was the key—a philosophy I continue in my own fitness studio today.

I became a weight loss and fitness junkie. As a matter a fact, I even spent three weeks during the summer between my junior and senior years of high school at Joe Weider's Bodybuilding Camp in Los Angeles. It was an amazing experience!

You'd think by the time I hit college I would have been an all-muscle, no-fat, Statue-of-David-looking young man. . . . Nope.

The thing that held me back—for a long time, and even at times today—was my all-or-nothing mentality.

I'm the type of person that can really dive into something. It's an awesome strength to have, when I wasn't letting "perfection be the enemy of good." This happened a lot early on, especially when it came to working out and eating.

Throughout high school, even though I never really stopped studying fitness and bodybuilding, I didn't always practice it. I'd either be "on" or "off." Workouts would take a backseat when I'd throw myself into whatever I was most passionate about at the time. It was a recipe for up-and-down results, frustration, hormone imbalances, and a messed-up metabolism that would make results even harder to achieve later in my life.

College offered a fresh start. I was excited to dive into fitness, and even I imagined myself owning my own community gym like the All American. I couldn't wait to attend all the science-related classes like exercise physiology, biomechanics, and advanced neuromuscular physiology. The college I chose had an awesome gym and hosted an annual National Physique Committee (NPC) bodybuilding competition that was for students only. I was so ready to learn and train!

Unfortunately, my freshman year did *not* reward me with a Greek god's physique. Instead of a slab of muscle, I packed on a bloated belly and a saggy chest.

I remember thinking at the time, *How could that be? I was training my butt off and eating a virtually no-fat diet.*

Looking back, I recognize that there were two key things working against me:

1. *The low-fat and no-fat crap that I was eating.* I was a big-time victim of the '90s fat-free craze, especially frozen yogurt. And all the carb-loading I did with pasta, and the

chemicals I'd top it with to give it some no-fat flavor. So bad!

2. *Stress!* I was one of the hardest working guys in the gym. I always felt like the underdog so I'd try to out-train everyone. I was overtraining!

When freshman year failed to improve my body, I worked even harder the next year. My sophomore year is probably when I did the internal damage to my body that still plagues me today.

Regardless, I signed up for my first bodybuilding competition that year. Because of weight classes and the excess weight I gained "bulking up," I had a long road before the competition. But I was determined and willing to work as hard as I had to and stick to my diet 100 percent.

I lost more than fifty pounds in fourteen weeks!

Now, that might sound awesome, but let me tell you, *it was not.* It took a super-low calorie diet and hours in the gym (sometimes three workouts per day) to achieve that kind of weight loss, which included the hard-earned muscle that I had gained the year prior.

Sure, I was shredded on stage, but that was short lived. I gained twenty pounds back in less than a week after the show and ultimately ended up almost right back where I had started fourteen weeks earlier. Looking back now, I can admit how bad I actually looked—I was super-skinny at 5'10", 148 pounds, with a 29" waist. It was not healthy *at all.*

You'd think after all that I would have finally learned my lesson. . . . *Nope.* I competed again the following year. I did make adjustments to both my training and nutrition plans to make them more realistic. As a result, I competed twenty pounds heavier while being almost as lean. But did I maintain my results this time? *Of course not.* All or nothing.

Eventually, I finished school and entered the workforce. I wound up doing what most newly degreed and certified personal trainers do: I gave up my dream of owning my own facility and got a personal training job at a big-box gym.

I learned a ton about personal training, program design for weight loss and fitness, and how to run an effective business. I was even named the most valuable trainer for one of the biggest health club chains in the country, became a top manager, and started training the trainers and managers for the whole company.

However, I became increasingly frustrated with corporate life. My own fitness began to deteriorate as I climbed the ladder, and I found myself losing sight of why I got into this business in the first place—*to help people look, feel, and perform their best in and out of the gym.* It wasn't long before I was at my all-time highest weight and feeling like crap about myself, not to mention often becoming ill.

That's when I decided to take a *quantum leap.*

I started my business in 2009 and became my first client. I started applying to myself the latest and greatest in exercise, nutrition, supplementation, rest and recovery, and stress management.

With Janell's help, I have been able to transform my body and live a truly healthy lifestyle—I haven't had a cold since spring of 2010! I still struggle some with the "all-or-nothing" mentality, but fortunately I've learned to "manage my minimums" (something Janell teaches) and stick to a plan that I enjoy and works well for me. I'm able to maintain a healthy body and mind. I'm much happier, too.

The lessons you're going to learn in this book are the culmination of our own research and experience with ourselves and thousands of others. What started as a boot camp in the park with seven people has grown into The Transformation Club, serving hundreds of clients locally and thousands more online. I'm truly happy and grateful to share this information with you. I know it will dramatically decrease the learning curve for you and get you the results you're looking for.

WHY WE DO WHAT WE DO

Simply put, we want to *transform* lives.

We believe people want to be healthy; they just lack awareness and they don't know how to navigate the endless amounts of marketing, propaganda, and, quite frankly, bullshit that has littered the industry.

We're here to clear the path and guide you along the way to achieving your better you.

While most fitness businesses are consumed with amassing memberships and sales, we are consumed with changing lives for the better.

We spend our resources learning about exercise, nutrition, stress management, rest, and recovery so that we can deliver better products and services that produce positive changes in the lives of the people we work with. That is how we attract *and* retain more members and customers, a fundamental *must* for any fitness business to survive— we just approach it from the other end—*results first.*

Our mission is to educate, motivate, and inspire you to become the very BEST version of YOU.

JOIN OUR COMMUNITY OF FRIENDS IN FITNESS

We invite you to join our Facebook Group—FREE Tips & Strategies to Lose Weight & Feel Great—at www.facebook.com/groups/FREELoseWeightFeelGreat/.

You can also join our free newsletter at www.TheTransformationClub.fitness.

We truly hope you enjoy reading our book as much as we enjoyed writing it. We know when you follow the program outlined, you *will* achieve your transformation goals.

HAVE FAITH & TAKE ACTION!®

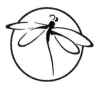

how to get the most out of this book

This book is filled with valuable, life-changing content. That's why we want to take a minute to give you an overview of the layout and how to best use it.

PART 1—THE MIND-SET PROGRAM

We begin with mind-set because *it is extremely important.* Access to information, regardless of how useful it, is worthless if you're not in the right frame of mind. This is something both of us have experienced ourselves. It's like reading a book for the second time—the information didn't change, you did. Where you are in your life and what your mind-set is strongly affects how you perceive and use information. It's critical to shed light on your mind-set and help you get into the right frame of mind to learn and apply the information and programs in this book.

PART 2—THE NUTRITION PROGRAM

The fact remains that *you can't out-train a bad diet!* As much as some would like to, you can't eat poorly and then just exercise the "bad" calories off. Besides, you'll soon learn that weight loss is *not* about calories in vs. calories out. This book is about *far more* than weight loss. In fact, when you follow the plan in this book, weight loss and maintaining a healthy weight is simply a positive side effect.

PART 3—THE TRAINING PROGRAM

Here you'll discover a fun, realistic approach to working out that doesn't consume your schedule or require hours of really boring exercise—like being stuck to an elliptical for hours each week.

PART 4—THE LIFESTYLE PROGRAM

Remember, this book is about *transformation* and becoming the BEST version of YOU. This part of the book features a series of chapters covering all the things that are often overlooked when it comes to a transformation program. Your transformation needs to be about more than just weight loss and sculpting a fit physique. To be the BEST version of YOU, you must be *happy, healthy,* and *fit.*

GETTING STARTED...

Though you're ultimately going to get the most value from this book by reading it from cover to cover, we also understand that you may already be focused and ready to get started *right now!* We certainly don't want to discourage that "get-it-done" attitude. If you're ready to jump in with both feet, skip ahead to Part 2 to get started on the supportive nutrition meal plan or Part 3 to get started on your first set of workouts.

As you work your way through your first week of eating and training, we urge you to come back to Part 1 to ensure that you are in the perfect mind-set to succeed.

One other thing: for live, ongoing education and support, be sure to join our Facebook group, FREE Tips & Strategies To Lose Weight & Feel Great.

Good luck, and remember to *HAVE FAITH & TAKE ACTION!*®

PART 1

THE MIND-SET PROGRAM

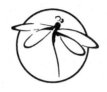

chapter 1

IT'S ALL IN YOUR HEAD

Quite frankly, if you don't get this part down, nothing else matters. Let's be clear—it's not like you can't get results without the right mind-set. You can begrudgingly follow the exercise and nutrition programs outlined in this book and get amazing results, but that's not the point. This isn't just another book/program that you suffer through to lose weight.

The book is titled *The Transformation Book* for a reason. The purpose of this book is to set you up for *long-lasting* success. But what *is* success?

The best definition of success comes from the legendary Earl Nightingale. He said, "Success is the progressive realization of a worthy ideal."

According to the dictionary, **ideal** is defined as, "satisfying one's conception of what is perfect; most suitable." Let's make it a point right now to get any ideas of "perfection" out of our head.

Justin's mentor, Bob Proctor, had an even better way to look at an ideal—call it *"an idea you've fallen in love with."*

It's also important to discuss the word **worthy** because it can be misleading. Too often, we look at ourselves and say, *"We're not worthy of X. We don't deserve to be/have/do X."* That's a bunch of crap! You were born and that alone makes you worthy of any good you desire.

Bob Proctor also wisely said that what you're doing needs to be worthy of YOU. After all, you have one life, so if you're going to dedicate your resources toward something, it better damn well be *worthy of you.* We think that getting/staying healthy is a worthy ideal, one that is critical to becoming the BEST version of YOU, but ultimately that's for you to decide.

Next, let's talk about the term **progressive**. This one is pretty simple to understand. It's about doing a little more and getting a little better than you were before.

The only person you should try to be better than is the person you were yesterday.

Focus on progress, not perfection.

When it comes to progress and weight loss, you're going to have your ups and downs and plenty of plateaus. Be okay with that, learn from the "wins" and the "losses," and most importantly, be kind to yourself.

Lastly, **realization** is simply about getting results. That's why you're reading this book, right? Good! Because *that* is what we're going to help you do.

Our mission is to educate, motivate, and inspire you to become the best version of you. You'll soon discover that this is a never-ending process. There will always be more to learn and more to share with those you love. It's a beautiful journey.

Let's begin.

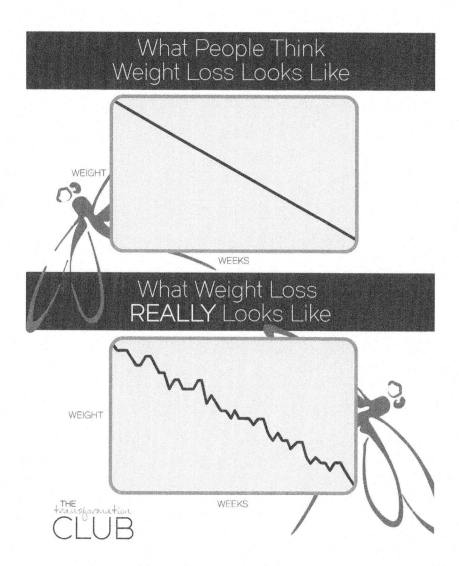

chapter 2

WHAT DO YOU THINK?

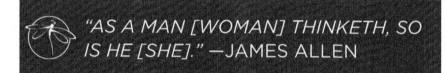

James Allen was a British philosopher and writer who is most famous for his inspirational books and poetry. The quote above comes from a marvelous book called *As a Man Thinketh* that Allen wrote at the turn of the 20th century. It is by far one of our favorite books, and a must-have for any library. Justin actually rewrote a version of the book, titled *As a Woman Thinketh*, because we work with so many women that we wanted to have a version that spoke to them.

We're going to share a couple passages here:

> The aphorism "As a woman thinketh in her heart so is she" not only embraces the whole of a woman's being, but is so comprehensive as to reach out to every condition and circumstance of her life. A woman is literally what

she thinks, her character being the complete sum of all her thoughts.

As the plant springs from and could not be without the seed, so every act of woman springs from the hidden seeds of thoughts, and could not have appeared without them. This applies equally to those acts called "spontaneous" and "unpremeditated" as to those that are deliberately executed.

Act is the blossom of thought, and joy and suffering are its fruits; thus does a woman garner in the sweet and bitter fruitage of her own self-care.

Of all the beautiful truths pertaining to the soul which have been restored and brought to light in this age, none is more gladdening or fruitful of divine promise and confidence than this—that woman is the master of thought, the molder of character, and the maker and shaper of condition, environment, and destiny.

The body is the servant of the mind. It obeys the operations of the mind, whether they be deliberately chosen or automatically expressed. At the bidding of unlawful thoughts, the body sinks rapidly into disease and decay: at the command of glad and beautiful thoughts, it becomes clothed with youthfulness and beauty. The body is a delicate and plastic instrument, which responds readily to the thoughts by which it is impressed, and habits of thought will produce their own effects, good or bad, upon it.

Change of diet will not help a woman who will not change her thoughts. When a woman makes her thoughts pure, she no longer desires impure food.

If you would perfect your body, guard your mind. If you would renew your body, beautify your mind.

These words explain exactly how the mind/body connection works to bring about all things in your life. We suggest you reread these passages daily. In fact, we encourage you to write them out (there's power in that) and carry them with you at all times—read them a few times each day. You'll find new meaning in them as you go through your transformation.

SUCCESS STARTS HERE

Before we can begin to make changes and see results, we must first understand how our minds control everything we do. Just like every other part of the universe, the mind is governed by very specific laws. These laws are present and all around us.

Let's take the most obvious example: the universal law of gravitation. You could get into some serious trouble for ignoring or not being aware of this law.

For example, you are on the edge of a building and decide to walk off the edge to see what will happen. You would fall—without exception. The same law applies for everyone, even an infant who is completely unaware of the law. *Ignorance of the law does not change its effect.*

To maximize your success, you must become familiar with and work with these laws. If you ignore them, you will pay the price. If you work harmoniously with them, you will be richly rewarded.

Mind-set and personal development are subjects that we are fascinated with and have benefited greatly from studying. In this section, we're going to share what we have learned. We have also included pages of recommend resources at the end of the book for you to study further.

THE GREAT LAW—ENERGY IS

Way back in elementary school science class, we learned the law that everything is made up of energy—the same energy, as a matter of fact. Here are some everyday examples to consider.

Take your hand, for instance. Stop a moment and take a look at it. Go ahead and hold it up in front of your face. Do you realize that your hand is a mass of molecules all vibrating at a very high rate of speed? Stop a moment and think. The book you are holding and reading, the water you drink, and the food you eat—they are all energy. Since everything is made up of the same energy, then it goes without saying—everything that ever was, is, and will be has always been here. That's pretty deep.

Consider airplane flight for example. The ability to fly has always been here. It just took the imagination, will, and determination of the Wright brothers to make us aware of it—to offer proof to us that it can be done.

The fact remains, however, the laws that make these tools possible today have always been there. It simply took awareness to bring them about.

The same rules apply when it comes to making your body healthy and fit. All it takes is an awareness of key information and abiding by certain laws to make it happen. By tapping into this energy, we can do virtually anything we set our minds to do.

Bob Proctor has been called "the mentor of mentors." Much of the information we're sharing here comes from various programs and seminars of his we've participated in. If you're not familiar with Bob Proctor or his bestselling book, *You Were Born Rich*, check it out. If you open your mind to the information he shares, you will literally change your life.

Bob Proctor has been a success coach for over fifty years, but he became recognized globally after his appearance in the world-famous DVD, *The Secret.*

Now, let's be very clear on one thing when it comes to *The Secret*, which is really about the *Law of Attraction*, you can't just wish for a thing and make it appear. You can, however, get into the right mind-set to raise your awareness of the resources available to you and attract more of what you need to achieve your goals, but you still must *take action*!

We have taken this concept to heart and made it a core value of our business:

HAVE FAITH & TAKE ACTION!

"Faith is the ability to see the invisible—to believe in the incredible. That is what enables you to receive what the masses think is impossible."

—Clarence Smithison

"People are always blaming their circumstances for what they are. I don't believe in circumstances. The people who get on in this world are the people who get up and look for the circumstances they want, and if they can't find them, make them."

—George Bernard Shaw

We foster our members' faith and provide them with the tools and coaching they need to take action to achieve their goals. We motivate, educate, and inspire them to be the very best version of themselves.

SEEING WHAT'S RIGHT IN FRONT OF YOU

Sometimes there are things in our lives that no matter how many times we've looked at them, we overlook the obvious. Some of the principles that we are covering in this book may be hard to comprehend and challenge you to think in different ways. They will challenge you to shift your paradigm into a new way of thinking and acting.

We rely so much on our five senses that we have a hard time believing something's existence if it isn't proven through our senses. Yet, our senses can be blinded or deceived. Sometimes there are things that have been right in front of us all along that we have seen countless times throughout our lives, but only when they are shown to us in a different way are we able to finally see what has been "hidden."

I'm sure you've seen the classic two-image drawings where you can "switch" what you see.

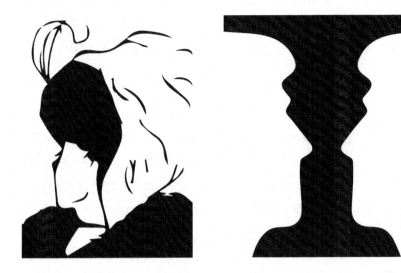

(L) Do you see the young lady or old woman? Both?
(R) Do you see a candlestick or two faces? Both?

Perception allows us to see things from different points of view. When you change the way you look at things, then you change the way they look to you. Perception is a powerful intellectual factor and a major contributor to the formation of your paradigms. Your paradigms literally control everything you do and, therefore, every result you get. In other words, what you see is what you get. How you view yourself will have a great impact on the results you get.

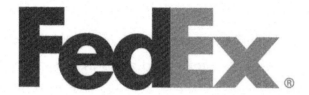

We've all seen this countless times throughout our lives, but did you ever notice the arrow in the FedEx logo, between the "e" and the "x"?

Don't feel bad. Most people never have. We certainly didn't until it was pointed out to us.

Open your mind to new ideas, and we promise you will open a door that will lead to amazing possibilities and personal greatness. When you begin to understand how your mind works and learn to tap into your "higher-self," you will manifest your healthy and fit body and realize it's been here all along.

 CASE STUDY: **MIND-SET MATTERS**

Learning about mind-set was a game changer for me. I have always struggled with my weight, and it seemed to me that the world would drop too much on my shoulders. I was shy and timid around people and would find comfort in food. I walked through my life feeling like a victim.

Desperately wanting to find something to help bring me happiness, I decided to get back into a workout routine and found Justin Yule.

My ah-ha moment came when Justin asked us to think about why we were in the workshop.

"What brought you here? It's not to lose weight," he said.

I remember driving home that night in tears, thinking about how I never felt good enough or worthy. That was my decisive moment. As I lay in bed that night, I walked myself through all those hard times and I rewrote my history. I stopped seeing the hardships and began to see the good, the beautiful, the fun, the love, and the happiness.

I learned that I am in control of my life, I am in control of how I react and how I deal with situations as they come up. I was able to see that I was getting in my own way, that I was blocking myself from success. Those key components helped me to learn that food is not meant for comfort, it's meant for fuel. I also realized that I am worthy—I don't need to hide—and that it's up to me to bring my own happiness and success. I lost seventy pounds and gained so much vital self-esteem and confidence.

—Shanna Ballsrud

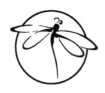

chapter 3

THOUGHTS & THINGS

The law of vibration states that everything vibrates and nothing rests. When you have conscious awareness of this vibration, it is called "feeling." Your thoughts control your vibrations and ultimately create your paradigms. Paradigms are essentially a multitude of habits developed by how you view the world around you—your perception—and they literally control everything you do.

For example, maybe your mother was overweight and you look a lot like her. So you assume that you will also be obese and cannot see yourself any other way. Therefore, the actions that you take (or don't take) cause you to be obese. The result reinforces the paradigm, and on and on the cycle continues.

"To ignore the power of paradigms to influence your judgment is to put yourself at significant risk when exploring your future.

*To be able to shape your future you have
to be ready to change your paradigm."*

—Joel Barker, *Paradigms*

When you are not feeling good about yourself, become aware of what you are thinking and instead think of something pleasant that makes you think outside of that paradigm. As difficult as it may be, hold this more positive image on the screen of your mind and block out the negative thoughts. With the power of choice, you *can* change your thoughts and your feelings. You can move from a negative and unsuccessful mind-set to a positive and successful mind-set in a flash. It is important to understand—until your thoughts and mind shift to a more pure and healthy image, you will never be able to have the long-term success you desire when it comes to getting fit.

To be healthy and fit, you must think and act like a healthy and fit person!

UNDERSTANDING THE MIND

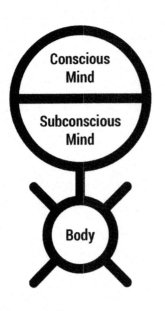

In 1934, Dr. Thurman Fleet came up with the stick person drawing as a way to help explain the workings of the mind. Essentially, we all think in pictures and (for most of us) having a picture of something will help us better understand it. For example, when you think of your car or your house, a picture is immediately projected onto the screen of your mind. When you think of your mind, what picture do you get?

Fleet's stick person consists of three parts: the *conscious mind, subconscious mind,* and *body.*

Your conscious mind is your "thinking mind" and it decides your attitude and level of success (or failure).

We are constantly bombarded by thoughts throughout the day. Studies have shown that upward of sixty thousand thoughts enter our mind each day! You have the ability to accept or reject any idea; *you* choose your thoughts. These ideas either originate in the conscious mind or they can be accepted from an outside source. The problem is that most of us are not thinking and the majority of those ideas are passing right through the "conscious filter." Once we accept the idea (good or bad), it is immediately impressed onto the subconscious mind.

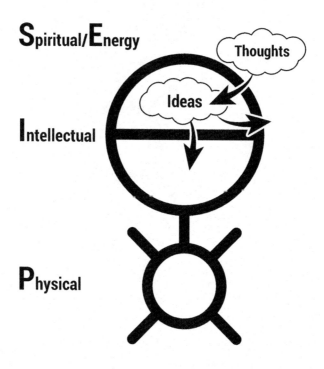

Unlike the conscious mind, the subconscious mind has no ability to reject ideas. It operates in an orderly manner. Your repeated, accepted, conscious thoughts become fixed ideas that express themselves without any conscious assistance until they are replaced by new ideas or paradigms. Understand that your paradigms literally control you. The good news is you can filter what enters your subconscious mind, thus forcing a paradigm shift.

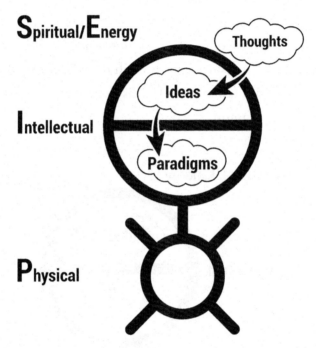

Your subconscious mind knows no limits except those that you consciously choose.

Your body is the material medium that is the instrument of your mind—or "the house you live in," as Bob likes to say. The thoughts or images that are consciously chosen and impressed upon the subconscious mind are what move your body into action. The actions you are involved in determine your results.

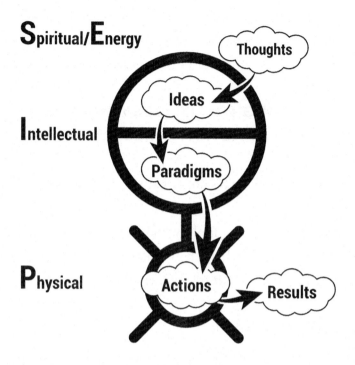

Let's give an example of how all this works.

A child is raised by obese parents. She is brought up in a sedentary lifestyle eating fattening foods. She naturally becomes out of shape. In school, she may be picked on and left out in gym class. Over time, she sees herself as fat and nonathletic. Once she defines herself this way, the paradigm has formed.

Naturally, with this paradigm she does not engage in physical activities and consistently eats unhealthy and fattening foods. The result of all this, of course, is a fat and unhealthy adult. This result continues to reinforce the old paradigm thus guaranteeing more and more of the end result: obesity.

Is she obese because of her genes or is she fat because of the actions she's taken, which were dictated by her paradigm, which was built from ideas that were fixed into her mind?

The thoughts you choose create the image you hold. The image you hold controls the feelings you have. The feelings you have cause the actions you take. The actions you take control the results you get.

THOUGHTS › IMAGES › FEELINGS › ACTIONS › RESULTS

So, you see, *you do* become what you think about, but you still have to act!

If you want to be a healthy and fit person, start acting like a healthy and fit person. That's how you will become a healthy and fit person. Essentially, "fake it till you make it!"

BETTER YOUR BEST

This statement is another of our business's core values. Here's what it means to us.

One of the most basic laws of life is "create or disintegrate." Nothing remains the same. You're either improving the quality of your life or you are taking away from it. We continually focus, both personally and professionally, on doing a little bit more and being a little bit better.

Cybernetics is the study of control and communication in machines to regulate or reach an end goal. Essentially, a cybernetic mechanism is a device that regulates a machine to achieve an end result.

For example, a thermostat is a cybernetic mechanism. Its job is to maintain the temperature of a room. If the goal is to keep the room at seventy-two degrees, then the thermostat will turn the air conditioning unit on or off as the temperature changes.

The autopilot on an airplane is another example of a cybernetic mechanism. Its job is to keep the plane on course so that the passengers arrive safely at the correct destination.

Cybernetics / *The study of control and communication in machines to regulate or reach an end goal*

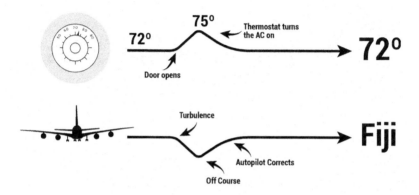

Psycho-cybernetics looks at the cybernetic mechanism inside us and how it relates to our potential. Pick up a copy of *Psycho-Cybernetics* by Maxwell Maltz for a deep dive. His concepts have influenced many psychological methods of training elite athletes. Maltz explains the mind–body connection as the key to success in attaining personal goals.[1]

Maltz became interested in why setting goals works. He learned that the power of self-affirmation and mental visualization techniques use the connection between the mind and the body. He specified techniques to develop a positive inner goal as a means of developing a positive outer goal. This concentration on inner attitudes is essential to his approach, as *a person's outer success can never rise above the one visualized internally.* Let's apply the idea of psycho-cybernetics to achieving a weight loss goal.

---

1   Maxwell Maltz, *Psycho-Cybernetics* (TarcherPerigree, 2015).

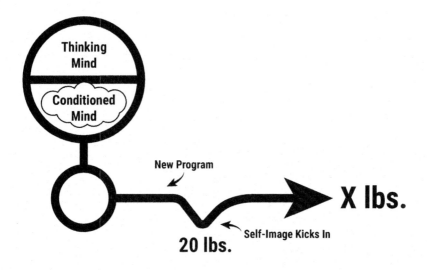

Right now you are *programmed* to weigh a certain amount. You weigh that amount because that is the idea you hold in your mind and you are conditioned to behave in such a way to bring about that result. If you were to change the behavior by starting on a proper exercise program, you will inevitably lose weight. For this example, let's say you lose twenty pounds. At some point, this change creates a "disturbance." It's not part of your normal programming. As a result, your self-image kicks in. Your conditioned mind is so tuned into the weight that you have been that it literally halts your progress and changes your behaviors to bring you back to its comfort point.

In the end, you ultimately gain the weight back. This cycle of weight loss and weight gain will continue *until* you change the image in your mind.

When you begin to see yourself at that desired weight, then and only then will you be able to move into action to achieve it *and maintain it*.

Watch Justin explain psycho-cybernetics and how it relates to your success at www.TheTransformationClub.fitness/ stickperson.

STEP UP TO SUCCESS

Your present results are a direct reflection of your current level of thinking and the ideas you hold in your mind. They operate on the same "frequency." Your goal exists on a higher frequency. The only way to achieve your goal is to raise your level of awareness. You must think and create ideas that operate on the same level of frequency as your goal.

"Both success and failure are the offspring of thought."

—Napoleon Hill

GETTING STARTED . . .

Take some time to really think about and answer the following questions. Write down your answers in a journal or in your smartphone.

- What is your health and fitness goal? Why?
- How will you feel when you achieve your goal?
- Do you believe you are worth it?
- What are paradigms, and why is understanding them so important in achieving your goal?
- What is your perception of yourself right now?

- How does your perception of yourself affect achieving your goal?

- What would you like your perception of yourself to be?

- What can you begin doing today to program your subconscious (conditioned) mind to move you into action to achieve and maintain your goal?

PART 2

THE NUTRITION PROGRAM

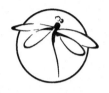

chapter 4

ALL CALORIES ARE *NOT* CREATED EQUAL

In our opinion, the *biggest* nutrition myth of all time is that *all calories are created equal.* The myth that fat makes you fat is right up there, too.

You have been made to believe that the key to losing weight and being healthy is to simply *eat less.*

Well, how is that working for you? We don't ask that question to be rude but rather to really have you ask yourself, "Is what you are doing right now with your nutrition working for you?"

When it comes to how you fuel your body, the *quality* of food is very important.

If you are thirsty, you wouldn't stop to drink water from a muddy puddle, because the issue isn't just about quenching your thirst. You understand and know that the quality of the water you drink matters. The solution isn't to "*drink less water,*" it's to "*drink better quality water.*"

The solution to today's obesity epidemic isn't to eat *less* food; it's to eat *higher-quality* food.[2]

When you fuel your body with quality food, the quantity tends to naturally take care of itself. However, there may be a few situations when tracking the amount of quality calories you are taking in would be appropriate and beneficial.

One of those situations is if someone is potentially undereating. It may be hard to believe, but this happens a lot! Another situation when tracking calories for a brief time would be beneficial is if you have specific, realistic goals that you are still having difficulties achieving after optimizing training, quality of calories, sleep, stress management, and recovery.

WHY COUNTING CALORIES DOESN'T WORK

Calorie counting doesn't work because different types of calories work differently inside your body. Lean proteins, vegetables, and healthy fats send different signals to your body than sugar, trans fats, and processed foods.

In his book *Why We Get Fat*, Gary Taubes talks about the twenty-calories-per-day theory.[3] If you overeat by just twenty calories per day starting at age twenty-five, says Taubes, you would gain twenty-one pounds in a decade. If you rely solely on counting calories, you would need to have 99.2 percent accuracy, and let's face it, no one can do that!

It's not counting calories that controls your metabolism but rather *your hormones.*

---

2   Jonathan Bailor, *The Calorie Myth* (New York: Harper Collis Publishers, 2013), 62.

3   Gary Taubes, *Why We Get Fat: And What to Do About It* (New York: Alfred A. Knopf, 2010), 58.

Counting calories is based on the assumption that the human body works like a balance scale, where it's all about managing calories in vs. calories out. It's just not that simple! A better approach is to eat foods that keep you satisfied, do not spike blood sugar, provide the body with nutrients, and cannot be easily converted to body fat.

In his book *The Calorie Myth,* Jonathan Bailor refers to this as eating "SANE" calories. SANE is an acronym for Satiety, Aggression, Nutrition, Efficiency.[4]

SANE calories heal your hormones such as insulin and leptin, prevent overeating, and lower your set point (the weight your body easily maintains).

Satiety

Satiety is the capacity of calories to make and keep you full. Have you ever noticed how you can easily eat a plate full of pasta? Imagine trying to do that with a plate of broccoli. You'd have to force feed yourself and you'd wind up uncomfortably stuffed!

Harvard researchers have found that the amount of protein in food affects the signals to our brain that tell us if we are hungry or full. It also affects our short- and long-term satiety hormones. When more calories are coming from protein, more "full" hormonal signals are sent to the brain.

To increase satiation, focus on foods that contain high amounts of water, fiber, and protein. When a food contains more water and fiber, you generally end up staying fuller longer. Vegetables provide both fiber and water; they are very satiating. However, protein also matters.

When you eat food that provides more satiety, you get too full for low-quality food.

---

4   Bailor, 64.

Aggression

The more *aggressive* a calorie is, the faster it will increase the level of glucose in your bloodstream. In turn, the hormones that affect fat storage are negatively impacted.

When blood sugar spikes in the body, insulin (a hormone secreted by the pancreas) rushes in to clear it from the bloodstream and transport glucose (broken down carbohydrates) into your cells. However, insulin is not on or off in your body. Instead, it is secreted in either a trickle, stream, or flood, depending on what you eat. If the pancreas has to secrete lots of insulin over time, it can overwork the system, leading to cells becoming insulin resistant, potentially leading to type 2 diabetes.

Eating foods that are high in water, fiber, and protein helps to control the insulin response in your body. You will then lower your risk for chronic diseases (heart disease, diabetes, and stroke) and will store less body fat.

Nutrition

Your body needs nutrients from food to carry out basic functions and metabolic processes and to be healthy. The amount and quality of nutrition affects your metabolism and whether or not your body is burning or storing fat and building or burning muscle.

Many overweight and obese individuals are actually undernourished versus overnourished.

When you eat low-quality *inSANE* foods, your body will continue to call for nourishment (more food) regardless of whether or not you met your daily caloric need. You continue to have food cravings and wind up overeating because your body is looking for the nutrition that it still requires.

It is important to consider nutrients relative to calories. If you eat 250 calories worth of nonstarchy vegetables, you would receive about forty-six grams of fiber. To get the same amount of fiber from whole grains, you would have to eat nearly two thousand calories worth of whole-grain bread. Eating whole-grain bread to get more fiber is like eating zucchini bread to get more vegetables.

Foods that provide many nutrients per calorie are nonstarchy vegetables, seafood, high-quality meats, low-fructose fruits, and nut/ seeds. Foods that provide very few nutrients per calorie are processed foods and sweets.

A food's nutrient profile largely depends on water, fiber, and protein. When you eat more water, fiber, and protein packed food, you get more essential nutrients and will avoid overeating or over-whelming your body with excess glucose.

When you consume foods that pack a lot of nutrition, your body will receive all of the nutrients that it needs and it will automatically regulate your appetite (and weight) without a struggle.

Efficiency

Efficiency has to do with how efficiently you convert calories to body fat. Counterintuitively, the more inefficient calories, the better (less likely to be stored as fat). Fiber and protein are entirely inefficient.

Fiber is not digested by the body and therefore can never be stored as body fat. Protein is five calorie-burning steps away from body fat. It takes five to ten times more energy to digest proteins than it does to digest fats or carbohydrates. That means you actually burn several calories in the process of protein digestion!

Calories that come from starch, on the other hand, are more than twice as efficient at becoming body fat than are calories from protein.

When you eat high-quality foods, you avoid overeating due to high *satiety*. Calories are released into your bloodstream slowly and trigger a small insulin release thanks to low *aggression*. Your body benefits from a number of essential *nutrients* from high-quality nutrition. You burn a lot of calories during digestion thanks to low *efficiency*.[5]

 # WHY WE DON'T COUNT CALORIES

Counting calories creates a mind-set of restriction and limitation. Your focus is on what you can't have rather than on nourishment, adding value, and improving food quality. When your brain perceives deprivation, it wants to rebel, be bad, and break the rules.

Counting calories doesn't take food choices into consideration. You can get two thousand calories from healthy meals spread over a day, or you can get it from a large latte and a couple of scones. Which is a better choice? When you focus on food quantity (number of calories), instead of the quality of your food, you are bound to make poor decisions.

Counting calories is inaccurate. The calorie counts on food package labels are often wrong. Calories are simply a measure of energy. They don't account for the way our bodies digest, absorb, and use this energy. Researchers estimate that even meticulous calorie counting can be up to 25 percent off. That

---

5   Bailor, 66–83.

means if you try to eat 2,000 calories, even if you do it "perfectly," you could be eating anywhere between 1,500 and 2,500 calories.

Counting calories is a pain in the butt. Unless you have a food scale and you meticulously weigh and track every morsel of food that goes into your body, you have no idea how many calories you are actually consuming.

Counting calories doesn't focus on building habits. The best way to achieve and maintain a healthy weight is to practice the habits that will lead to your *outcome goal.* Calorie counting is a very small (and time-consuming) part of the big picture. Most people try to lose weight by counting calories, which is exactly why they ultimately fail. The truth is, you can get the body you desire without ever being that meticulous. We don't count calories and you likely don't need to, either.

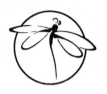

chapter 5

HORMONES & WEIGHT LOSS

Calories from lean proteins, vegetables, and healthy fats work differently in your body than calories that come from sugar or processed carbohydrates. *Remember SANE calories?*

Instead of focusing on calories, you must focus on eating the right types of food to turn on your fat burning and turn off fat storing.

This is where your hormones come into play. The hormone that has been talked about for the last fifty to sixty years in regard to storing fat is insulin.

Insulin is the regulator of fat metabolism. It puts fat into fat tissue and suppresses fat mobilization. In order to get fat out of fat tissues, you must make your insulin work for you, not against you. The bottom line: when insulin is secreted or chronically elevated, fat accumulates in the fat tissue. When insulin levels drop, fat escapes from the fat tissue and the fat deposits shrink.

We secrete insulin primarily in response to the carbohydrates in our diet. Insulin is not on or off in our body, it is secreted in either a trickle, stream, or flood based on what we eat. By eating foods that keep your insulin levels low and steady, you help regulate your appetite and control cravings. If insulin levels are high, your body will not use fat for a fuel source and has a hard time stabilizing blood sugar.

Once insulin has done its job after a meal, only then can your body enter a true fat-burning state. Our metabolism is not meant to handle eating and snacking all day. When a person eats a snack, it raises insulin, no matter what that snack is. It is a myth that you need to eat six times a day to keep your metabolism going!

When insulin is secreted, it shuts off fat-burning mode and allows triglyceride levels to stay too high for proper leptin function, reducing proper leptin entry into the brain. This can cause excessive food cravings, an unstable energy level, poor head function, and unproductive sleep.

Hormonal imbalance starts when you overconsume the wrong types of carbohydrates. Carbohydrate intake drives insulin and insulin drives fat accumulation. You positively impact insulin by managing your blood sugar.[6]

As of late, another important hormone has been discovered. That hormone is leptin, and in order to achieve your fat-loss goals, leptin must be balanced. **Leptin is the most powerful hormone in the human body.** It is the commander in chief of energy use—no other hormone tells leptin what to do.

Leptin is what gives your body the full signal after you eat a meal.

---

6   Byron J. Richards, *The Leptin Diet* (Minneapolis, MN: Wellness Resources, 2011), 34–36.

Leptin follows a twenty-four-hour pattern where levels are highest in the evening hours and peak late at night. Leptin also sets the timing for nighttime repair, as well as coordinating the function of melatonin, thyroid hormone, growth hormone, sex hormones, and immune system function to carry out restorative sleep. This hormone burns fat at the greatest rate at night but only if you allow it to do so. In a person with normal leptin function, the brain gets the signal that they are full and do not require any more food in the evening. However, those with leptin problems or leptin resistance never get a proper full signal (until they overeat), and they are driven by subconscious urges to eat from the time dinner is over until the time they go to bed.

If leptin is not working properly you may experience: fatigue, depression, irritability, inability to focus, poor metabolism, faulty immune function, problems extracting energy from food, high cholesterol, high blood pressure, diabetes, or obesity, and the list goes on and on. Most people can relate to at least a few of these symptoms.

Leptin is made in fat cells. If leptin is working you will have a healthy metabolism, and your appetite will be held at bay. If leptin is low, you will have a slower metabolism, and your appetite will be stimulated.

So, in theory, if someone has a lot of fat stores they should also have a lot of leptin and have a high metabolism and not be hungry. Quite the opposite is true: most of the time, overweight or obese individuals have a slow metabolism and are hungry all the time.

Why? Because the brains of overweight or obese individuals have become resistant to leptin and, therefore, their brain thinks leptin is low. This will slow down their metabolism and increase their appetite. Insulin resistance and leptin resistance mean that the hormones are not communicating efficiently in response to food. Therefore, a person has to overeat in order to get enough leptin into the brain to get a full signal.[7]

WHAT CAUSES LEPTIN RESISTANCE AND HOW DO YOU MANAGE IT?

Caloric restriction, insulin and blood sugar issues, stress, overeating, increased triglycerides, and fructose (*specifically high-fructose corn syrup*) all contribute to leptin resistance. Whenever insulin is negatively impacted, leptin is negatively impacted as well.[8]

The first way you manage leptin is by managing insulin. Insulin is *increased* when you eat too many carbohydrates (*especially simple carbs*). You manage insulin by managing carbohydrate intake.

Another way to manage leptin is to decrease stress. If cortisol is dysregulated, then you will have blood sugar issues, despite a supportive nutrition plan that contains the appropriate amount of carbohydrates. Cortisol is the hormone secreted when your body is under stress.

Always including protein at breakfast and not overeating will also help you to control leptin. If you are overweight, always try to finish a meal when you are less than full. It takes ten to twenty minutes for the brain to catch up and signal the body that you are full. Eating slowly can assist with this.

When all of these signals are working properly, you feel full longer. You no longer have uncontrollable cravings for sweets. And your fat is burned for fuel, helping you to achieve and maintain a healthy weight.

---

7   Richards, 8–14.
8   Richards, 14.

HOW DOES STRESS AFFECT HORMONE BALANCE?

You can manage this dangerous dance between blood sugar and insulin by what you eat or through a stressful situation. Stress can come from external stressors, such as running late for an important meeting, or stress can be internal, an overgrowth of bad bacteria or a gut pathogen. Cortisol is our stress hormone: chronically elevated cortisol levels increase blood sugar because our body is in "fight or flight" mode and thinks we need the energy to run from the stressful situation.

This state of elevated blood-sugar levels can contribute to insulin resistance and promotes belly fat. Unfortunately, many of us find ourselves in stressful situations where this physiological response happens several times a day.

MEAL TIMING

Meal timing is key in managing blood sugar and hormones, especially leptin. There are two strategies for doing so:

1. *Never ever* eat after dinner.

2. Eat three to four meals a day.[9]

NOTE: *Allow at least two hours between your last meal of the day and the time you go to bed. Space dinner and breakfast out so that there are at least eleven to twelve hours in between.*

Three to four hours after a meal, blood-sugar levels naturally begin to drop because insulin is done doing its job of transporting calories into cells. Now our bodies can use stored calories for energy.

---

9   Richards, 43.

The drop in insulin signals the pancreas to produce glucagon. Glucagon's job is to maintain blood sugar in absence of food. Glucagon then signals the liver to release glycogen (stored glucose) in order to maintain blood sugar levels. *In a sense, your body is getting a snack, just not from food.*

Between meals, about 60 percent of fuel will come from sugar stored in the liver, and under the signal from glucagon the liver will burn 40 percent fatty acids. Triglycerides from fat stores are now being used as fuel. This starts happening three to four hours after a meal and continues until the next meal. This is fat-burning time. As long as energy levels are maintained, the longer a person stays in fat-burning mode, the more fat they will burn. Snacking or eating too often confuses leptin, and sooner or later this will catch up with you. In order to avoid leptin issues in the evening, you must properly manage leptin during the day.[10]

It will take some time and practice to figure out the best meal timing for you and your lifestyle. How many meals you eat each day and the timing of those meals will change and fluctuate depending on what is going on in your life. If you are working out more, you may need to increase the frequency of your meals and pay more attention to the timing of your meals pre- and post-workout to get the most out of your training.

If you are in a time of high stress, you may need to eat more frequently to help stabilize your blood sugar and support your adrenal glands. Our point in talking about this is to make you aware that, just like other things in your life, what you need nutritionally is *not* static. What you do at one point in your life to support your health and lose weight may not work for you at another point.

---

10   Richards, 36–38.

That's because your body and the circumstances of your life have changed, and your goals may be different. Your training, nutrition, and lifestyle support will then be different as well. It is important to be clear on what your goals are, what is realistic for your life right now, and then formulate a plan around that.

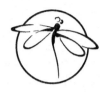

chapter 6

INFLAMMATION—FIGHTING THE FIRE WITHIN

Inflammation is the first response by the immune system to infection or irritation. There are actually two types of inflammation: one is necessary and the other can be detrimental to your health. Inflammation can present in any of the following ways: redness, heat, swelling, pain, and dysfunction of the organs involved.

Acute inflammation is needed to help heal acute trauma, abrasions, broken bones, or acute invasion of a foreign substance, such as bee venom from a bee sting. This is the inflammation we can see and feel.

Acute responses to stress are important because they keep the body from doing further damage to the injury or wound by promoting pain and swelling all around the injured areas. We want and need this type of inflammatory response to happen in the body in order to heal.

Chronic inflammation is an ongoing, low-level inflammation, invisible to the human eye. It usually occurs as a response to prolonged acute inflammation or repetitive injuries. Chronic inflammation can and will eventually lead to tissue destruction.

This is the type of inflammation that we may not even know is there but which has much more severe consequences than some swelling or bruising. When our bodies can no longer regulate inflammation, *"Houston, we have a problem!"*

"Unfortunately, chronic inflammation typically will not produce symptoms until actual loss of function occurs somewhere. This is because chronic inflammation is low-grade and systemic, often silently damaging your tissues over an extended period of time. This process can go on for years without you noticing until a disease suddenly sets in."

—Dr. Mercola

Researchers are finding more and more evidence linking chronic inflammation with chronic diseases, such as, cardiovascular disease, cancer, Alzheimer's disease, autoimmune diseases, and asthma. Chronic inflammation in the heart can cause heart disease; in the brain, dementia and Alzheimer's disease; and in our fat cells, obesity.

Research also links obesity with inflammation. Being overweight promotes inflammation—which promotes obesity. It is a vicious cycle. *More than 50 percent of Americans are inflamed and don't even know it!* Anything that causes inflammation can cause you to gain weight, and any weight that you gain can cause more inflammation.

SOURCES OF INFLAMMATION

The Standard American Diet (SAD) of sugar, processed food, trans fats, gluten, alcohol, etc., combined with lack of exercise, environmental allergens, infections, stress, and toxins increase inflammation in our bodies.

Inflammation comes from the sugar we eat, high doses of the wrong kinds of oils and fats in our diet (omega-6 & omega-9 vs. omega-3), hidden food allergies/sensitivities, lack of exercise, chronic stress, hidden infections, and our fat cells.

Believe it or not, your own fat cells—especially the ones around your middle—are often one of the *biggest* sources of inflammation. Fat cells (adipocytes) produce hormones such as leptin, which reduces appetite; resistin, which makes you more insulin resistant; and adiponectin, which makes you more insulin sensitive and lowers your blood sugar. Fat cells also produce the hormones estrogen, testosterone, and cortisol, as well as inflammatory molecules.

Fat cells are busy controlling appetite, hormonal balances, and inflammation. The molecules produced by your fat cells wreak havoc on your metabolism by increasing inflammation, increasing your appetite, slowing fat burning, and increasing stress hormones.[11]

These molecules exist in abundance when your system is out of balance from too much stress, sugar, trans fats, or exposure to toxins, allergens, or infections.

Eating poor-quality foods (sugar, trans fats, processed foods, etc.) that don't fit our evolutionary needs will trigger your body to release inflammatory messages that prevent critical parts of your metabolic system from working, thus crippling your metabolism and causing you to gain weight.

---

11   Mark Hyman, *Ultrametabolism, The Simple Plan for Automatic Weight Loss* (New York: Atria Books, 2008), 133–134.

The fat around your middle makes a "fire" in your belly that spreads throughout your system by sending out these inflammatory messenger molecules throughout your body. Fire or inflammation anywhere in the body creates more fire in the belly, creating a vicious cycle of inflammation, oxidative stress, and metabolic changes that leads to weight gain, metabolic syndrome, or prediabetes, just to name a few.

The solution is to get into a healthy cycle—getting rid of inflammation helps you lose fat, and losing fat helps you get rid of inflammation.

Refined Seed Oils

A major source of inflammation in our diets comes from refined seed oils. Consuming these oxidized refined oils can deplete your body's antioxidants and increase inflammation inside the body.

Refined seed oils include: canola oil, soybean oil, peanut oil, cottonseed oil, corn oil, sunflower oil, safflower oil, vegetable oil, flaxseed oil, and grapeseed oil.

These oils are found in:

- margarines

- salad dressings

- mayonnaise

- sauces

- chips

- popcorn

- frozen entrees

- baked goods

- and just about any other processed food

These oils are also used in almost all restaurants because they are *very* cost-effective. Due to the high-heat process used to extract oils from these seeds, the delicate polyunsaturated fats and nutrients they contain are damaged. These oils are usually rancid by the time they hit grocery store shelves. Plus, once they do arrive in stores, they sit under bright lights for who knows how long.

Refined oils will also skew your dietary ratio of omega-6 to omega-3 fats in the wrong direction. A high dietary ratio of omega-6 to omega-3 is associated with more inflammation. It is estimated that the SAD has *fifteen to twenty times* as many omega-6 to omega-3; the ideal ratio should be close to 1:1.

To improve your health and reduce inflammation, decrease your total polyunsaturated fat intake and improve your omega-6 to omega-3 ratio by avoiding refined oils. The two most effective ways to do this are by reducing how often you eat out at restaurants and avoiding packaged and processed foods and salad dressings.[12]

Food Sensitivities

Food sensitivities can also be a source of inflammation. By doing a detox/elimination diet, such as Janell's 21-Day Detox Challenge, you can identify foods that you are eating that could be the cause of chronic inflammation and health and weight issues.

---

12   Chris Kresser, "How Too Much Omega-6 and Not Enough Omega-3 Is Making Us Sick," *Let's Take Back Your Health* (blog), May 8, 2010, https://chriskresser.com/how-too-much-omega-6-and-not-enough-omega-3-is-making-us-sick/.

21-DAY DETOX CHALLENGE

The 21-Day Detox Challenge is a comprehensive program based around eating whole foods and eliminating common inflammatory foods. It is designed to help you identify how certain foods are affecting you physically, mentally, and emotionally. Through education, grocery shopping lists, recipes, and daily emails, you are set up for twenty-one days of success. Common results of this program include but are not limited to: more energy, sleeping better, weight loss, less joint pain, and clearer skin. For more info or to sign up, visit www.21daydetoxchallenge.info.

The idea of an elimination diet is to give your body a break from common food allergies/sensitivities and to see if you lose weight and your symptoms get better/disappear. The type of food sensitivity I am referring to has a delayed response; it can be anywhere from a few hours to a few days after ingestion.

Many people have food sensitivities and don't even know it! They are unaware of the connection to the symptoms (tired, crabby, depressed, headaches, joint pain, etc.) they are experiencing to what they ate twenty-four to seventy-two hours ago.

Food sensitivities are more common than you may think—one in three people will experience a food sensitivity in their lives. Many of these sensitivities go undiagnosed, leaving individuals to suffer from symptoms that are never traced back to their diet.

GLUTEN FOR PUNISHMENT

In the last three and a half years, Janell can count on one hand how many times she has knowingly eaten gluten. One of those times was when we were in Chicago. We wanted some deep-dish, traditional Chicago pizza. So Janell ate a few pieces, along with a big salad to get in some veggies. Prior to this particular incident, Janell chose to avoid gluten because it left her feeling bloated, constipated, and unpleasant.

What she hadn't noticed in the past was her mood after eating gluten. This time there was no way both of us weren't going to notice the effects on her mood. We had the pizza on our last night in Chicago and we were driving more than six hours home the next day. *For the next forty-eight hours, Janell was cranky, depressed, unmotivated, tired, and quite frankly unpleasant to be around.* She knew those feelings all too well because she used to feel like that *all the time*! At one point, Janell was taking medication for anxiety and depression.

Since she hadn't felt like that in so long, it was *very* clear that it had to do with something she had eaten. *Gluten and refined carbohydrates were the culprits.*

Eating foods that you are sensitive to puts constant stress on your digestive system and immune system and compromises your vitality. Loss of vitality can lead to depression, lethargy, and brain fog.

The most common foods that people are sensitive to are:

- gluten (the protein found in wheat, barley, and rye)

- dairy (especially cow milk)

- soy

- corn

- wheat

- eggs

- nuts

- nightshades (eggplant, tomatoes, white potatoes, peppers, and any spices that include peppers)

We can develop food sensitivities when the lining of our gut and the balance of normal gut flora get damaged from poor diet, stress, medications, infections, or toxins. This is referred to as *leaky gut*.

Leaky gut is when the tight junctions that line our guts get pulled apart by one or more of the prior items mentioned. Undigested food particles can then get into our system and our body will treat these particles as foreign invaders. The immune system will create antibodies against them and this immune response will increase inflammation in the body.

Symptoms of leaky gut include but are not limited to:

- fatigue

- food sensitivities

- GI problems (bloating, abdominal pain, diarrhea, constipation)

- autoimmune conditions

- joint pain

- headaches and migraines

- skin problems (hives, eczema, rashes, acne)

- concentration issues (foggy head)

- asthma

- depression

- anxiety

- behavioral problems

- fertility problems

- underweight or overweight

- adrenal fatigue

- liver problems

- nutritional deficiencies

Since the immune system can become overtaxed, these inflammatory compounds can get out into the bloodstream and affect nerves, organs, connective tissues, joints, and muscles. Hence the variety of symptoms caused by food sensitivities. If you are sedentary, have poor sleep patterns, eat a Standard American Diet, and/or have high stress levels, you can almost be sure that your gut lining is starting to pull apart and food particles will start to leak through.

NOTE: *An individual can have food sensitivities but have zero symptoms related to the gut and GI system. Your immune system can start to recognize the undigested food particles/proteins as similar to other proteins that make up your thyroid or cerebellum, for instance. You may start to experi-*

ence symptoms that are far removed from what someone may equate to food or the GI system.

 ## GOING WITH YOUR GUT

The health of your digestive system directly impacts your overall look, feel, and physical performance. When it comes to optimizing your digestion, it really does pay to listen to your gut.

You may not realize it, but digestion begins in the mouth; while chewing, enzymes from saliva mix with food to break down carbohydrates. Proper chewing prepares food for digestion. Chewing too quickly and swallowing prematurely leave food particles too large for stomach acids to break down. Large food particles make it difficult for the small intestines to absorb food molecules and extract nutrients.

Food then enters the stomach and mixes with additional enzymes and hydrochloric acid (HCL). The ability to properly digest food in the stomach is dependent upon having adequate production of HCL and digestive enzymes. From the stomach, digestion continues in the small intestines.

The small intestines are roughly twenty-five feet long. Digestive enzymes from the pancreas and bile from the liver are released into the small intestines to aid in the digestion of foods. Once receptors have digested the food, it's sent through the portal vein to the liver for processing. Unwanted or indigestible food particles are sent to the colon for final processing before being excreted out of the body.

The large intestine, otherwise known as the colon, is five to six feet long. Trillions of bacteria live here, some of them friendly, and some not. Unfriendly bacteria can promote gas, bloating, constipation, or other GI distress. Friendly bacteria aid in healthy digestion. The optimal ratio is 85 percent friendly to 15 percent unfriendly. However, many people today have closer to 85 percent unfriendly and only 15 percent friendly. Because friendly bacteria stimulate movement of the colon, this prevents constipation and makes the environment unfavorable for unfriendly bacteria.

Digestion is a complex process and if it doesn't start out well, there will likely be other issues further down the chain. Some common symptoms of poor digestion include gas, bloating, headache, burping, reflux, fatigue, muscle and join ache, and constant hunger. Chronic poor digestion even leads to leaky gut syndrome, food intolerance, and a stubborn paunch belly.[13]

---

13   Paul Check, *How to Eat, Move, and Be Healthy!* (C.H.E.K. Institute, 2004), 215–216.

Gluten

Gluten is one of the most common food sensitivities a person can have. *It is linked to more than fifty-five diseases.*[14] Gluten is actually a protein that is found in wheat, rye, barley, spelt, and some oats. It is extracted from these grains and used in other foods to add texture and protein, as well.

Gluten is highly addictive. You have receptors in your brain that are affected by gluten much the same way that opium affects them. This is one reason why gluten can be so difficult to eliminate from your diet. Gluten is known to cross the intestinal barrier, either intact or partly digested, and can disproportionately feed the bacteria in the gut, leading to gut dysbiosis. It also stimulates the release of zonulin, which acts directly on the tight junctions in the gut; this causes them to open and allows the contents of the gut to leak out. Once gluten has leaked out, it interacts with the immune system of the gut.

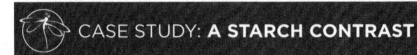

CASE STUDY: **A STARCH CONTRAST**

My favorite foods growing up were all white, starchy, refined carbs. My absolute favorites were bagels with cream cheese and pasta with a hefty dose of Parmesan cheese.

I had dealt with chronic stomachaches, bloating, indigestion, diarrhea, and cramps for as long as I could remember. It's sad to admit, but that was my "normal."

---

14   Richard J. Farrell and Ciarán P. Kelly, "Celiac Sprue," *N Engl J Med* 346, no. 3 (2002), 180–188.

It wasn't until I was in college and was diagnosed with mononucleosis, recurring strep throat, a tonsillectomy, and major fatigue—all in just a few short months—that we began to get to the bottom of my GI discomfort.

My body was essentially in crisis mode. My mom had heard about a local doctor and made me an appointment. The doctor ran a series of nutrition sensitivity tests that discovered I was gluten, dairy, soy, and corn intolerant, along with being very sensitive to preservatives, petroleum, and parabens.

I remember getting the results and crying. This was my whole diet and now I had to stop eating almost everything I liked! This was years ago, before gluten-free eating had taken off, and it was difficult to find alternatives.

It's been a very enlightening few years. I have learned not only the immediate and long-term signs my body is not happy with something I ate but I have discovered new cooking methods, friends, and likeminded individuals/groups (like The Transformation Club) and a newfound sense of empowerment to advocate for myself. I truly think that removing gluten was the first step in peeling back the layers of dysfunction I had accumulated over the course of my life. My asthma has improved, and the brutal allergies I used to have in the spring and fall are nearly nonexistent now.

I have grown to appreciate my body for what it is and feels like on the current day. Am I fueling properly?

Am I feeling lethargic? Am I feeling emotional mood swings? How is my stress? I never thought that first doctor appointment would lead to a total body awareness journey.

—Allie Fancher

Who Needs to Avoid Gluten?

If someone has been diagnosed with celiac disease, they have a condition in which the body experiences an immune reaction when gluten is consumed. The result of this condition is damage to the inside of the small intestine. This, in turn, impairs the absorption of important nutrients.

There is also a condition known as gluten sensitivity. Gluten sensitivity is a disorder of the immune system that has a wide range of manifestations throughout the body and brain. This reaction to gluten is less severe and less damaging to the small intestine than celiac disease, but physical symptoms are still present, such as nutritional deficiencies, gastrointestinal difficulties, headaches, joint pain, and a wide array of other symptoms.

When gluten is consumed, the immune system responds by producing inflammation, and this inflammation damages tissues throughout the body. The immune response from gluten is delayed (from ten minutes to two days) but long lasting. Many people who have gluten sensitivity seem to have zero symptoms, which can make the diagnosis and avoidance more difficult.

It's not just those who have a diagnosed sensitivity to gluten who are removing it from their diets. Many healthy people are eliminating gluten because they want to reduce processed carbohydrates in their diets and eat more whole foods. The vast majority of breads, pastas, pizzas, baked goods, and processed foods are full of gluten and carbohydrates. When you eliminate gluten from your diet, your carbohydrate choices now come in the form of whole foods: vegetables and fruits. Eliminating gluten from your diet also decreases inflammation and toxins in the body, both of which can increase our risk for disease down the road as well as hinder our progress to lose weight.

 CASE STUDY: **MY BELLY KNOWS BEST**

I never had food allergies growing up. Living on a farm with nine brothers and sisters, I couldn't afford to be too picky if I wanted to fill my stomach. But when I turned forty several years ago, I went through a six-week cleanse with a friend. I cut out everything but lean meats, fruits, and vegetables.

At the end of the six weeks, I felt clean and healthy and also dropped eight pounds. My doctor suggested I add in the old foods one at a time. Coffee and dairy were no problem, but when I had pasta, I instantly felt as if I had a rock in my belly! I was nauseated, bloated, and gassy; it took two days for my digestive system to feel normal again.

I went to a gastroenterologist and had some testing done. It was a relief to learn I did not have celiac disease, but otherwise, there were no definitive results. My doctor said I probably had sensitivity to gluten and that I should avoid it. It was tough to hear—it seemed impossible to avoid something that was seemingly present in everything on the table.

I'm still not sure why this sensitivity developed or if it's always been there and just got worse over the years. All I know is that I feel sick if I eat it, so I avoid gluten whenever possible. I have missed fresh bread and pancakes for breakfast, but my belly knows best.

Several years ago it seemed hard to avoid gluten, but now there are plenty of gluten-free alternatives and it's easier to select meals that are wholesome and delicious, both at home and at a restaurant.

—Charlotte Swanson

GLUTEN-FREE PROCESSED FOODS

When removing gluten from the diet, people take a few different approaches. Some will simply make the switch from gluten-containing products to gluten-free counterparts, while neglecting whole, unprocessed foods. Others consume a combination of both natural and packaged gluten-free foods. Another approach would be to consume solely naturally gluten-free foods.

If someone notices once they choose to go gluten free that their symptoms are not improving or they are not achieving their weight loss goals, it is likely that they are consuming too many gluten-free packaged foods.

With the explosion of interest in gluten-free products, food manufacturers have stepped up the production of baked goods, breads, pizzas, etc., that look, taste, and feel like traditional gluten-containing foods, but are, in fact, gluten-free. From cinnamon rolls to pastas to muffins, there is a gluten-free option to satisfy nearly any craving you might have.

This is good news for those who need alternatives, but it is also bad news because it is easy to mistake gluten-free for carbohydrate-free and healthy. The two are not the same! It is *very* important to keep in mind that processed food is processed food whether it is gluten-free or not.

Gluten-free products often have even more refined carbohydrates than do their gluten-containing counterparts. Any processed foods, gluten-free or not, lose a lot of their nutrients during the refining process. In order for gluten-free flours and products to be manufactured, grains and starches such as rice, potatoes, corn, and tapioca are used. While these things are free of gluten, they are still highly processed and refined and, therefore, can cause a spike in blood sugar higher than that of their whole-grain counterparts.

Carbohydrates are found in many other grains and foods and are often present in significant amounts in gluten-free products. It is tempting to think that because a cracker or brownie is gluten-free you can eat as many as you want. You can't. Those crackers and brownies are likely to be very high in carbs and contain just as much or more sugar than a gluten-filled counterpart.

Eating too many carbohydrates (especially refined carbohydrates) for your activity level will limit your ability to lose weight and will likely result in weight gain. This is because too much insulin (fat storage hormone) production to regulate blood sugar spikes from these high-sugar, high-carbohydrate foods.

Your best defense is to be informed. Know what you are eating. Before you eat a gluten-free product, read the label. Check the ingredients, the carb and sugar count.

DAIRY

Dairy is the other most common food sensitivity. Everywhere we turn it seems milk is pushed as the perfect food. Long touted as necessary for proper growth for both children and adults alike, milk and many milk products are seen as innocent when it comes to health.

Unfortunately, research is mounting that indicates that dairy is not as good for you as it was once thought.

One of the biggest problems with conventional dairy is where it is coming from and how it is processed. Most cows on conventional farms are given antibiotics and growth hormones, all of which we ingest when we consume conventional dairy.

Janell grew up on a dairy farm and limits her consumption of dairy because of how her body reacts to it. She actually does much better on goat dairy then she does with dairy from cows. The conventional milk and dairy products that you purchase at the grocery store are very different than when Janell's mom got milk right out of the bulk tank on the farm for her family's consumption. This raw milk contained live enzymes and nutritional value. The milk you buy in the grocery stores has been stripped of most of its beneficial properties.

Another thing to consider when it comes to dairy is that not all dairy is created equal. You may not experience any adverse effects from a small amount of raw cheese or grass-fed yogurt, but drinking milk may not work for you. Or like Janell, you may be able to tolerate dairy from goat or sheep much better than from cows. This is why it is important to *eliminate all* dairy for at least three weeks and then reintroduce one type at a time to determine if you are experiencing symptoms as a result.

Common symptoms include but are not limited to: acne, excess mucous production, insulin imbalances, and gastrointestinal problems.

There are several reasons why some people have a hard time tolerating dairy and may experience adverse side effects after consuming it. Among the top reasons are:

- They do not contain the proper enzymes to digest the lactose, which is the sugar found in dairy products. As you age, your ability to digest lactose may decrease.

- They can't break down one or both of the proteins found in dairy. The two proteins are whey and casein. Most individuals cannot properly digest casein. That is why some people like Janell can tolerate a high-quality whey protein powder but experience symptoms, such as acne, when they have too much cheese.

NOTE: *Not all whey protein powders are created equal! For example, Justin does fine with one certain whey protein powder but has gastrointestinal stress with most others. You want to look for one that has very few ingredients and does not contain soy or artificial sweeteners like sucralose.*

If you discover that you can tolerate dairy without any adverse side effects, then choose high-quality dairy that is raw or grass-fed. For example, if we are going to choose to eat ice cream, we make sure it is high-quality ice cream from grass-fed cows!

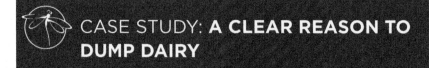

CASE STUDY: A CLEAR REASON TO DUMP DAIRY

I discovered that I was lactose intolerant after I gave up dairy for twenty-one days and then reintroduced it into my diet. Almost immediately after drinking milk and eating cheese again, my entire digestive system changed for the worse. I was bloated and I had gas. Within a couple of days I had acne again. I've been off dairy for a few years now and I feel amazing. I have more energy, less fatigue, and clear skin. I also had the unexpected benefit of losing weight and keeping it off.

—Julie Stuart

CALCIUM DEBATE

Perhaps the biggest reason many people drink milk is because they believe that it offers a calcium boost that insulates them from developing osteoporosis. On the surface, this appears to make sense, until we stop to consider that *the United States is one of the biggest consumers of dairy products in the world and we also have one of the highest rates of osteoporosis in the world.* If all that calcium was protecting our bones, we should be seeing lower rates of this disease. In fact, in a study of ten countries, a higher consumption of calcium was associated with a higher risk of bone fracture!

What Is Going On?

Our bodies prefer to be in a state of slight alkalinity. When that preferred state is changed and becomes more acidic, the body will do what is necessary to buffer the acid and return to an alkaline state. This is done by pulling salts and minerals from the bones to neutralize the acid.[15]

When milk is consumed, the proteins in it create an acid environment in your body. Your body responds by pulling buffering agents from your bones. Over time, this results in bones that become weaker, not stronger.

There are much better sources of calcium that will deliver benefit to your bones, with none of the dangers that dairy products bring.

These include:

- broccoli

- dandelion greens

- collard greens

- kale

- quinoa

- chickpeas

- navy beans

- sesame seeds

- almonds

Let's be honest, breaking free from dairy and gluten can be hard. But if you keep your mind set on the benefits that await

---

15   Susan E. Brown, *Better Bones, Better Body* (New York: McGraw-Hill Education, 2000), 134.

you—less inflammation, stronger bones, better digestion, and better immunity—the work involved will seem easier.

 STRESS

Stress can dramatically increase inflammation! Relaxation and reducing stress can dramatically reduce inflammation. For more information about stress, be sure to read chapter 21.

TURN DOWN THE FIRE

There are many prescription and over-the-counter drugs that you can take to decrease inflammation. Most commonly are NSAIDS (nonsteroidal anti-inflammatory drugs) such as Ibuprofen or aspirin. It is likely that your symptoms will subside, but the root cause of the problem is *not* being addressed. Unless you get to the root of where the inflammation is coming from, you have simply postponed the inevitable. The fire is still there; it is just contained, at least for the time being.

Making changes in your diet, lifestyle, and exercise can and will reduce inflammation. What you eat and how much you exercise are the most important factors governing inflammation. A diet high in fiber nonstarchy vegetables, low-glycemic fruits, and omega-3 fats reduces inflammation and improves insulin sensitivity. Increasing fiber not only lowers inflammation but also C-reactive protein levels, which is an indicator of inflammation in the body.

One of the most important and powerful actions you can take when it comes to your diet is to eliminate all inflammatory foods (sugar, gluten, dairy, corn, soy) from your diet and notice how you feel, how you look, how you perform, and what happens to those nagging symptoms you were experiencing.

Lifestyle factors—such as appropriate exercise, proper restorative sleep, managing stress levels, engaging in positive interactions with others, getting in nature, and keeping a positive attitude—will all aid in cooling the inflammatory response in your body.

The good news is that you can *stop* chronic inflammation. It will require changes and shifts in your diet and lifestyle and it may also require some detective work to identify other potential sources of inflammation.

Sources of inflammation such as too much sugar, processed food, alcohol, or stress can be more obvious than sources such as food sensitivities, mold, medication, hidden infections such as viruses, parasites, or bacteria that don't cause immediate or obvious symptoms.

Decreasing and eliminating inflammation is not easy, but the results in your weight and health will be worth it!

FOODS THAT DECREASE INFLAMMATION

Omega-3 Fatty Acids

Omega-3 fats are one of the best things to incorporate into your diet to reduce inflammation. Omega-3 fatty acids are a group of fats found in a wide variety of foods, most famously in fish. Foods that are sources of anti-inflammatory omega-3 fatty acids include but are not limited to: grass-fed beef, wild caught salmon, flaxseeds, walnuts, sardines, cauliflower, and Brussels sprouts.

Nonstarchy Vegetables

Plants and nonstarchy vegetables, in particular, contain many anti-inflammatory phytonutrients. Eat seven to nine servings of non-starchy vegetables per day to ensure you are receiving enough of these healing nutrients. Nonstarchy vegetables are also low-glycemic, promoting healthy blood sugar regulation, which will ultimately decrease inflammation.

Nonstarchy vegetables include: artichoke hearts, asparagus, beets, broccoli, bok choy, Brussels sprouts, cabbage, cauliflower, bell peppers, carrots, celery, cucumbers, daikon, greens, tomatoes, spinach, snap peas, green beans, yellow beans, string beans, eggplant, jicama, kohlrabi, mushrooms, radishes, rutabaga, salad greens, squash, Swiss chard, turnips, water chestnuts, and onions.

Dark Chocolate

Dark chocolate contains phytonutrients called polyphenols. These are natural antioxidants and anti-inflammatory molecules that turn down the fire on inflammation. The dark chocolate you choose must be free of added saturated fats and rich in cocoa (70 percent or higher) and have only minimal amounts of sugar. A serving would be two to three ounces a couple times per week, not the entire dark chocolate bar at one time.

Herbs

Herbs that reduce inflammation include: capsaicin (from cayenne pepper), green tea, ginger, quercetin (fruit and vegetable rinds), turmeric (yellow spice found in curry), and cocoa.

TESTS FOR INFLAMMATION

In addition to the questions at the end of this section, there are also a few tests that can provide you with information as to the level of inflammation in your body. The C-reactive protein test is commonly known to assess cardiovascular risk, however, the C-reactive protein quantitative test measures for inflammation in the body. You may be able to get this blood test done through your doctor or you can directly order from websites such as http://requestatest.com. Keep in mind this is one measure; even though results may appear in the "normal" range, you still can't be sure there isn't any inflammation present somewhere in the body.

It is important that you take both test results and symptoms in account. Two common reasons that C-reactive protein may be elevated are metabolic syndrome or insulin resistance is present. Or it may be elevated due to some sort of reaction to a food (sensitivity, true allergy, or an autoimmune reaction).

Food sensitivity tests also offer information about what may be the source of inflammation in your body. These tests most often look for elevated antibodies (IgG) against specific foods, identifying if foods that you are eating are initiating an immune response and therefore increasing inflammation. A cheaper and often more effective way is to do an elimination/detox diet such as Janell's 21-Day Detox program.

You must understand how important it is to identify the sources of inflammation in your life. Once you have identified the sources of inflammation that are affecting your health and weight, start making changes to cool the fire.

"You don't lose weight and then get healthy,
you get healthy and then you lose weight."

—Janell Yule

Incorporate anti-inflammatory foods and herbs, exercise, and reducing stress through relaxation. Your weight will come down as you cool the fire of inflammation inside your body, and the rest of your health will improve at the same time.

 ## HOW INFLAMED ARE YOU?

YES NO

☐ ☐ Do you have a diagnosed autoimmune condition such as rheumatoid arthritis, Hashimoto's disease, type 1 diabetes, psoriasis, or celiac disease?

☐ ☐ Do you have skin issues (eczema, acne, rosacea, or rashes)?

☐ ☐ Do you experience excess mucus or get sinus infections?

☐ ☐ Do you experience joint pain?

☐ ☐ Do you get migraines or frequent headaches?

☐ ☐ Do you have food sensitivities?

☐ ☐ Do you experience high amounts of stress in your life?

☐ ☐ Do you drink three or more alcoholic beverages per week?

☐ ☐ Do you exercise less than twenty minutes three days per week?

☐ ☐ Are you overweight?

☐ ☐ Do you experience chronic digestive distress
(gas, bloating, constipation, or diarrhea)?

☐ ☐ Do you get more than one cold or infection
per year?

Add up the number of questions for which you answered yes.

0–3 = low inflammation

4–6 = moderate inflammation

7 and above = high inflammation[16]

---

16   Hyman, 130–131.

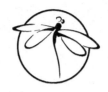

chapter 7

JUST EAT REAL FOOD

WHOLE FOODS

The food we eat is meant to nourish us physically, emotionally, and mentally and actively enhance our health and well-being. When we shifted our focus from, *"How many calories does X food have?"* to *"How does X food provide my body with nutrition?"* the choices we were making dramatically changed! We went from drinking diet soda and eating frozen dinners to eating wild salmon with roasted vegetables and drinking kombucha. Talk about a BIG difference!

The more you consume high-quality, high-nutrient-dense foods, the more sensitive your palate becomes. You enjoy food more, not less. And you are satisfied with smaller portions. If you choose foods that are delicious, full of nutrients, and the best quality you can afford, then you run out of room for the junk. But if you choose nutrient-poor, low-quality food, then you won't really feel satisfied physically or psychologically.

CASE STUDY: **THE REAL SECRET TO WEIGHT LOSS**

For me, pregnancy was a free-for-all when it came to food. After my first pregnancy I managed to lose most of the weight I gained. But with my second pregnancy, I ate whatever I wanted, whenever I wanted. After having my second son, the pizza, ice cream, and pasta weight remained. And this time, it wasn't going away. I didn't want to be in any pictures with my new baby or the rest of my family because I was embarrassed of how I looked. I always considered myself an average to thin person, so weighing 190 pounds was devastating. That wasn't me; it wasn't how my body was supposed to look. I knew I needed a big change. That's when Janell and Justin introduced me to this crazy "diet." Only eat *real* food! Yeah, it's not that crazy, it's just common sense. Only eat real food. If you can't pronounce it, don't eat it. If it wasn't living at one time, or from something that was, don't eat it.

So I cleaned out my fridge and pantry, only real food remained. I stocked my pantry back up with new foods. Each grocery trip ended with a cart full of produce and meats instead of cookies and chips and Lean Cuisines. I started cooking food instead of reheating premade convenience meals. I tried food I never had before and loved it. I have to be honest, eating this way does take work. It takes a lot of time and energy to plan out and cook meals. But to me, it was worth it.

This new way of eating, along with resistance training a few days a week, started to melt the pounds away. In less than six months, I lost fifty-five pounds. And the weight has stayed off. I don't have to yo-yo diet anymore, the scale doesn't go up and down like it used to. I give my body what it needs, and it stays healthy. To me, a real-food diet is how we were meant to eat. We weren't meant to eat all those convenient boxed, frozen, or premade meals. I love knowing that I am feeding my family the food their bodies need and teaching my children to eat healthy, delicious, *real* foods.

—Lindsay Belden

Learning to eat healthy isn't just about taking away the "not so good stuff." It's really more about adding more of the *good stuff—stuff that gives you more nourishment for your buck.* Whole foods deliver more value, nutrients, and nourishment to our bodies. They contain nature's medicine cabinet—a variety of phytochemicals and compounds that promote health.

Whole foods usually contain these chemicals and compounds in a form that we absorb and digest. *Whole foods contain these chemicals and compounds in the proportions that are appropriate.* There is no risk of overdosing on vitamins or minerals, unlike with supplements.

Whole food nutrients work together, not in isolation. Oftentimes, you need substance A to absorb or digest substance B. And often, A and B are in the same food. It's like the food evolved to be that way.

Whole foods are closest to their original form. You can expect to get the maximum nutrition possible, especially if those foods are fresh, seasonal, and local.

Whole foods match our hunger and fullness cues better. We are able to stop when we have had enough.

Whole foods taste better. Once our palate adapts, whole fresh food that is in season tastes so good while highly processed, chemical-laden food doesn't. It just tastes like chemicals.

 ## IS THIS A WHOLE FOOD?

Here are several questions to ask yourself about the food you are consuming.

- How is this food made?

- What's in it? (Or not in it?)

- Do I know what all these ingredients are?

- How does this food affect my body? How do I feel physically after eating it?

- Does this food physically nourish me? Does it add or subtract value?

- Is this the best available choice in my current situation?

- Do I find it easy or difficult to eat this food slowly, to 80 percent full?

COLOR THE RAINBOW

Eating a wide variety of vegetables and fruits of various colors will ensure that you get different phytochemicals into your body that help to ward off disease and stay healthy. Different nutrients are associated with the different colors of food.

Red: Contain nutrients such as lycopene, ellagic acid, quercetin, and hesperidin. These nutrients reduce the risk of prostate cancer, lower blood pressure, reduce tumor growth and cholesterol levels, decrease damaging free radicals, and support joint tissue in cases of arthritis.

Orange: Contain beta-carotene, zeaxanthin, flavonoids, lycopene, potassium, and vitamin C. These nutrients reduce age-related macular degeneration and the risk of prostate cancer, lower cholesterol and blood pressure, promote collagen formation and healthy joints, fight harmful free radicals, encourage alkaline balance, repair damaged DNA, and work with magnesium and calcium.

Yellow: Contain beta-cryptoxanthin and carotenoids lutein and zeaxanthin, which support intercellular communication, prevent heart disease, and reduce the risk of cataracts and age-related macular degeneration.

Green: Contain chlorophyll, fiber, lutein, zeaxanthin, magnesium, calcium, folate, vitamin C, and beta-carotene, which inhibit the action of carcinogens and promote healthy bodily function.

Purple & Blue: Contain phytochemicals such as anthocyanin and phenolics, powerful antioxidants that help reduce the risk of cancer, heart disease, and Alzheimer's, improve memory and cell communication, and slow the process of aging.

White: Contain beta-glucans, EGCG, SDG, flavonoids, alicoln, and lignans that activate natural killer B and T cells, support immunity, and balance hormone levels.[17]

If you *only* eat certain foods, you are missing out on nutrients that nourish your body and keep you free of disease. Challenge yourself to try a new vegetable this week and strive for lots of color in your diet.

SUPERFOODS

Superfoods are packed full of beneficial nutrients. These are the foods that give you the most bang for your buck. Eating these foods makes us healthier and adds value to our bodies.

For example, one cup of kale…

- has 206 percent of your daily requirement of vitamin A, 134 percent of your vitamin C, and a whopping 684 percent of your vitamin K;

- contains lots of trace minerals, such as copper and manganese;

- contains valuable phytonutrients, such as lutein;

- contains dietary fiber; and

- is anti-inflammatory.[18]

When you eat plenty of superfoods, there won't be much room for less optimal choices. Plus, you will benefit from a host of vitamins, minerals, good fats, protein, antioxidants, and other phytonutrients.

---

17   Juliann Schaeffer, 2008, "Color Me Healthy—Eating for a Rainbow of Benefits," *Today's Dietician* 10(11) (2008), 34.
18   Chris Gunnars, "10 Health Benefits of Kale," *Authority Nutrition*, https://authority nutrition.com/10-proven-benefits-of-kale/

Nutrient-Dense Foods to Add to Your Supportive Nutrition Plan

- **Wild Salmon**—best source of anti-inflammatory omega-3 fats. Aim for two to three servings of wild caught salmon each week.

- **Grass-Fed Beef**—packed with omega-3 fats and is one of the best protein and fat sources you can eat. Corn-fed beef is almost entirely stripped of omega-3 fats.

- **Free-Range Eggs** (especially the yolks)—naturally fed eggs will be full of vitamin D, omega-3 fats, and amino acids. Much like corn-fed beef, grain-fed chicken eggs are lacking in many of these nutrients. Free-range eggs contain a dark-orange yolk. This is where a large portion of the eggs' precious vitamins are.

- **Coconut Oil**—the most potent source of lauric acid and has high levels of MCTs (medium-chain triglycerides), which are antimicrobial and antiviral. MCTs help to increase the body's ability to process long-chain fatty acids—great news when you are trying to drop those last few pounds.

- **Liver**—the most nutrient-dense food on the planet. Because it is so nutrient-dense, you only need a few ounces. If you can't get yourself to eat liver, try a desiccated liver supplement instead.

- **Bone Broth**—a good source of minerals like calcium, phosphorus, magnesium, and potassium in forms that your body can absorb. It also contains glycine and proline, amino acids that are not found in significant amounts in muscle meat. Bone broth also contains gelatin, which can improve joint pain and sleep quality and enhance the quality of our hair, skin, and nails.

- **Fermented Foods**—improve our gut flora. Foods such as sauerkrauts, kimchi, fermented vegetables, and kombucha introduce live probiotics into your gut flora.

- **Sardines**—one can have more than 100 percent of your daily B12, 63 percent of your vitamin D, 24 percent of your B3, and 12 percent of your B2, as well as smaller amounts of every other vitamin except for C. Sardines also contain calcium, selenium, phosphorus, iron, magnesium, copper, and zinc.

- **Blueberries**—one of the most concentrated sources of antioxidants that nature has to offer. The deep blue color of blueberries is representative of their strong antioxidant properties. They are also said to help rehabilitate brain function.

- **Dark Chocolate**—cocoa contains a potent mix of antioxidants and flavonoids that boost cardiovascular health while fighting off high blood pressure. These flavonoids can also be very anti-inflammatory. The key here is moderation, have a small square of at least 80 percent pure dark chocolate and receive the benefits of this superfood.

It's pretty evident now that the quality of the calories you eat is far more important than the quantity. We are not saying that quantity *never* matters, but it is just more important that you start with changing the quality of your diet. You can surely overdo it with whole, healthy foods, but it is far less likely. One of the most common healthy foods we tend to see people overeat is nuts/nut butters. Focus on variety in your diet and you will be less likely to fall into this trap. Also, be sure to pay attention to the hunger, craving, and full signals that your body is constantly giving you.

Start by focusing on adding in as many whole foods, foods rich in color, and superfoods to your diet as you can. You will quickly start to see the benefits in how you look, feel, and perform.

EATING FOR THE SEASON

When you can, take advantage of farmers' markets and Community Share Agricultures (CSAs). Take time to explore your local farmers' market, see what is *in season* that week, buy fresh local produce, and then plan your meals around it. You just can't beat fresh, local produce!

There are plenty of benefits to eating in season. When produce is in season in your local area, the abundance of the crop makes it less expensive. Take berries for example. In the middle of January, you could pay $6 to $7 for a half a pint of fresh blueberries. But when berries are in season, you will likely find pints or even bigger containers for $3 to $4. It's the basic law of supply and demand, when crops are in season you are rewarded financially by purchasing what's in season. To enjoy all year long and to save costs, when certain fruits and vegetables are in season, buy extra and freeze them.

Plus, we all want the food that we eat to taste good! Especially our vegetables and fruits! When food is not in season locally, it's either grown in a hothouse or shipped from other parts of the world, and both will affect the taste. When crops are transported, they must be harvested early and refrigerated so they don't rot. Thus, they might not ripen as effectively as they would in their natural environment.

As a result, they don't develop their full flavor. For example, compare a dark red, vine-ripened tomato still warm from the summer sun with a winter hothouse tomato that's barely red. There is no comparison, the summer tomato's flavor is much more robust.

A VARIETY OF NUTRIENTS

According to Brian Halweil, author of *Eat Here: Reclaiming Homegrown Pleasures in a Global Supermarket*, "If you harvest something early so that it can endure a long-distance shipping experience, it's not going to have the full complement of nutrients it might have had."[19]

Transporting produce also sometimes requires irradiation (zapping the produce with a burst of radiation to kill germs) and preservatives (such as wax) to protect the produce, which is subsequently refrigerated during the trip.

Eat for the Season Year-Round!

- **In the spring**, focus on tender, leafy vegetables that represent the fresh new growth of the season. Think lots of green with Swiss chard, spinach, romaine lettuce, fresh parsley, and basil.

- **In the summer**, focus on light, cooling foods in the tradition of Chinese medicine. Foods include fruits, such as strawberries, apple, pear, and plums; vegetables, such as summer squash, broccoli, cauliflower, and corn; and spices and seasonings, such as peppermint and cilantro.

- **In the fall**, shift to more warming foods. The autumn harvest includes carrots, sweet potatoes, onions, and garlic.

19   Brian Halweil, *Eat Here: Reclaiming Homegrown Pleasures in a Global Supermarket* (New York: W.W. Norton & Company, 2004).

Focus on warming spices and seasonings, including ginger, peppercorns, and mustard seeds.

- **In the winter**, eat almost all warming foods. All of the animal foods fall into the warming category, including fish, chicken, beef, and lamb. Most of the root vegetables, carrots, potatoes, onions, and garlic are also warming.

Many regions have limited growing seasons, making it virtually impossible to eat locally and in season 100 percent of the time. *So what do you do?* The best possible scenario is to grow it and pick it yourself—that way you know exactly what went into growing those vegetables and can enjoy them at their peak the day they are harvested.

But if gardening isn't your thing, then visiting a local farmers' market weekly or joining a community-supported agriculture (CSA) farm is the next best thing. While it isn't always possible to purchase your seasonal produce locally, a good option is to purchase what's in season somewhere else. Hopefully that's close enough to minimize shipping time.

Determine what's in season right now and you will benefit from high-quality produce, packed with nutrition, at a lower cost. To find out what is harvested seasonally in your area, check farmers' markets near you and seasonal produce guides. Your taste buds, health, and body will thank you!

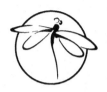

chapter 8

BUILDING A SOLID NUTRITION FOUNDATION

When a house is built, the first thing that happens is a solid foundation is poured. From there they build the structure, add walls, and so on. In this chapter, we are going to talk about building a solid foundation for your supportive nutrition plan and healthy lifestyle. It is important to build a solid foundation (~90 percent consistency) before you start worrying about the newest supplement or tracking grams of carbohydrates.

BEHAVIORS VS. OUTCOMES

If you want to lose weight, you can eat well, stay active, rest and recover, and manage stress. But you can't control what your fat cells are going to do. In other words, you can't control the outcome. However, what you can control is the behaviors that lead to the outcome you want.

So instead of setting and focusing on outcome goals, a better practice is to focus on behavior goals. Examples of behavior goals are: eating six to eight servings of vegetables per day or being in bed by 9 p.m. Behavior goals are things you do consistently and regularly. Behavior goals are small manageable tasks that are within your control. They are often things that you can do right now or in the near future.

Controlling behaviors effectively will lead to better outcomes.

 BASICS TO MASTER

- **Eat vegetables at each meal**. Your mom and grandma always told you to eat your vegetables. Nutritional science now backs up the importance of a diet packed with vegetables. Along with micronutrients, they contain important phytochemicals that are essential for optimal physiological functioning. Vegetables are full of water and fiber and provide an alkaline boost to the blood.

- **Eat protein at each meal**. It can be pretty difficult to look, feel, and perform at our very best without consuming adequate protein. Sources of protein include: eggs, beef, lamb, pork, chicken, turkey, fish and seafood, and high-quality protein powders. Women want to eat twenty to thirty grams of protein at each meal—the equivalent of about one palm-size portion. Men want to eat forty to sixty grams of protein per meal—the equivalent of about two palm-size portions.

- **Eat healthy fats daily**. Consuming healthy fats will optimize health, body composition, and performance. They keep us satiated and add flavor to our food. They are not something to fear but rather you should seek out nutrient-dense sources and incorporate them into your supportive nutrition plan. The key is to minimize and eliminate processed fats, particularly in the form of refined seed oils.

- **Carbohydrate timing.** If fat loss is your goal, eat veggies and fruits with every meal, and "other carbohydrates" only after exercise. You must earn your starchy carbohydrates. These are yams, plantains, sweet potatoes, beans, or rice. When we consume carbs post workout, they will get stored in the liver and muscles first as glycogen for future activity, before they are stored as fat.

EAT VEGETABLES AT EACH MEAL

When it comes to vegetables, we often hear, "*I don't like vegetables.*" Well, it's time to put on your "big boy" or "big girl" pants and continue to try different vegetables and ways to prepare them. Janell was the pickiest eater and *never* ate vegetables, until she realized that if she was going to improve her health and achieve her fitness goals, she needed to figure out how to eat more vegetables.

Vegetables are nutritional powerhouses and contain essential vitamins and minerals, along with phytochemicals and antioxidants. They are truly the foundation of every high-quality, health-promoting nutrition plan. If there was one thing that would dramatically reduce your risk of chronic disease and help you shed body fat, eating at least six to eight servings of vegetables per day would be it.

> **NOTE:** *A serving of vegetables is two cups of salad greens, one cup of raw, or half a cup of cooked.*

When you eat more vegetables, you can eat more food, with more valuable nutrients. Because vegetables are packed with fiber and water, you will feel fuller, healthier, and more energetic.

Nonstarchy vegetables include: asparagus, bok choy, romaine lettuce, red cabbage, red peppers, radishes, tomatoes, carrots, yellow peppers, artichokes, broccoli, green cabbage, cucumbers, kale, green peppers, Swiss chard, asparagus, green beans, Brussels sprouts, celery, lettuce, snap peas, spinach, zucchini, eggplant, cauliflower, jicama, mushrooms, onions, rutabaga, and spaghetti squash.

Starchy vegetables include: beets, butternut squash, winter squashes, parsnips, turnips, and pumpkin.

Often, the barrier for people to eat more vegetables is simply learning how to cook them. Start to become adventurous! When you know how to choose, prepare, and cook vegetables, it gives you confidence and variety.

Vegetables can be prepared by roasting, steaming, grilling, or baking. This week, try a new way of preparing your vegetables. One tip to get in more vegetables is to use them in soups or stews.

FOCUS ON ADDING, NOT SUBTRACTING

Pick one of the following strategies for adding in more vegetables this week:

- Add greens to your shakes and smoothies.

- Make soup or stew in your slow cooker with vegetables.

- Add cut-up vegetables such as mushrooms, spinach, peppers, onions, or broccoli to your scrambled eggs.

- Have raw vegetables washed and cut up for snacks; carrots and celery work great.

- Eat a big salad with dinner.

EAT PROTEIN AT EACH MEAL

Aside from water, proteins are the most abundant molecules in our bodies. Proteins are made up of thousands of smaller units called amino acids.

The benefits of protein include:

- Helping to build and repair almost every tissue in our bodies, including muscles and bones. They can also contribute to luscious hair, skin, and nails.

- Along with amino acids, proteins are essential for producing adequate enzymes, hormones (especially the ones that make us happy and relaxed), neurotransmitters, and antibodies.

- Supporting our immune system.

- Boosting our metabolism and helping us to maintain a healthy weight.

- Helping to keep us feeling fuller longer. When you eat enough protein, eating to 80 percent full gets a lot easier.

- Eating a solid serving of protein with breakfast will help to control your appetite all day long.

Protein sources include but are not limited to: grass-fed beef, organic free-range chicken, chicken sausage, organic free-range turkey, organic pasture-raised pork, nitrate-free sausages or bacon, wild Alaskan salmon, cod, scallops, white fish, shrimp, tuna, bison, ostrich, elk, venison, organic free-range eggs, and whey protein powder, vegetarian (rice, pea) protein powder.

Complete sources of protein come from animals and provide our bodies with all of the necessary amino acids (building blocks of protein).

Incomplete sources of protein are plant sources; a couple of different sources need to be eaten together in order to provide the body with all of its amino acid needs. Beans would be an example of an incomplete source of protein.

How Much Protein Do I Need?

The amount of protein each individual needs will vary depending on body size, activity level, and weight loss and fitness goals. A good place to start for an adult looking to build muscle and strength is .6 to .9 grams of protein per pound of bodyweight per day. This works out to about 90 to 135 grams of protein daily for a 150-pound person.

If you are eating protein at each meal, three to four times per day, the amount you need per day is likely being met. Ladies, you need to eat more than one or two eggs for breakfast! One egg contains about seven grams of protein; therefore, you want to eat three eggs and some bacon or sausage on the side.

When you are looking at your plate, you want about a palm-size portion of protein (or a portion the size of a deck of cards), then fill the rest of your plate with nonstarchy vegetables and possibly some starchy carbs.

Ways to incorporate more protein into your supportive nutrition plan:

- Prepare extra protein on the weekends or for dinner to have as a leftover the next day.

- Hard-boil a dozen eggs on the weekend.

- Add a quality protein powder to your morning smoothie.

- Have a small serving of lunch for an afternoon snack to ensure protein intake.

EAT HEALTHY FATS DAILY

Fat is important for normal cell functioning and nervous system function. It supports satiety, is necessary for normal hormone production, and is a great long-lasting source of energy. Fat provides your body with consistent energy by not triggering an insulin release like sugar and processed carbohydrates. One of the biggest nutrition myths of all time is that dietary fat is bad for our health. Which is why we have a whole chapter dedicated to fat!

There was a time when we embraced foods that contained natural fat, but somewhere along the line we started to believe that dietary fat equated body fat. We avoided foods high in saturated fat and cholesterol in hopes that it would prevent disease and improve our health.

Avoiding fat isn't the answer! Despite having more calories per gram than carbohydrate or protein, studies show that high-fat (and low-carbohydrate) diets actually lead to more weight loss than low-fat diets. This is because a diet based on real, unprocessed whole foods allows us to control and manage our hormones, which leads to weight loss.

 ## TYPES OF FATS

▫ *Saturated fat*

- Aim for a third of total fat intake from these fats.

- Include animal fats (eggs, grass-fed dairy, meats, grass-fed butter, ghee).

- Coconut oil is made up of medium-chain fatty acids, which yield 25 percent fewer calories per gram than most other fats. The fat in coconut oil is digested and metabolized differently than other fats. It can even help you lose weight. The fats from coconut do not get bundled up into lipoproteins, seeking out fat cells to make bigger. Instead, they go straight to the liver where they are used for energy. The medium-chain fatty acids found in coconut also help your body blaze through slower-burning long-chain triglycerides.

- *Monounsaturated fat*
  - Aim for a third of total fat intake from these fats.
  - Include olive oil, nuts and nut butters, avocado.
- *Polyunsaturated fat*
  - Aim for about a third of total fat intake from these fats, focusing on the omega-3 fats.
  - Include flax seeds, fish oil, nuts and nut butters, wild salmon.

When cooking with oils and fats, especially at high heats, **saturated fats are generally a better choice**. Grass-fed butter or ghee, coconut oil, red palm oil, duck fat, and beef tallow are wonderful options. Unsaturated fats are less stable and more prone to becoming trans-fats at high heat. Unhealthy oils that are heavily processed and should be avoided include: soy, corn, safflower, cottonseed, and canola oils.

DON'T GO NUTS!

It can be very easy to overeat nuts, after all they are delicious and versatile. Most nuts and seeds that we consume are high in fat, which makes them high in calories. The fats found in nuts are generally healthy fats, so they're beneficial but in appropriate amounts.

When eating nuts and nut butters, pay attention to the following:

- Keep your portions small, about ten whole nuts or about one tablespoon of nut butter.
- Eat plain raw nuts, not flavored, and/or salted ones.

- Be aware of any potential intolerance symptoms.

- Notice if eating nuts/nut butters is a "trigger habit" for you. In other words, if one handful or spoonful leads to ten more.

Natural fats that occur in properly raised animals, avocados, nuts and seeds, coconut, and olive oil are a part of a healthy supportive nutrition plan. Remember, fat is not the problem. It's the wrong types of fats coming from refined seed oils and trans fats in processed foods that are the problem.

Including fat at each meal is important because fat will keep you full and satisfied longer. When you have appropriate amounts of fat in your diet you actually end up eating fewer total calories because your body has the nutrition that it requires and your taste buds are satisfied.

WHAT IS MY CARBOHYDRATE TOLERANCE?

When it comes to carbs, there are so many *rules* that it can make you crazy! Remember your body always knows best. Tune in to what it is telling you with physical sensations.

- How do you feel when you eat a lot of sugar or processed foods?

- How do you feel when you eat six to eight servings or more of high-fiber veggies?

- How do you feel when you eat more healthy fats and protein?

- How do you feel if you choose a banana instead of a candy bar?

It's important to notice and name how your body feels when you make certain food choices. This is an important practice in putting together your personal supportive nutrition plan.

- Do you have consistent energy for your workouts?

- Are you recovering well?

- Are you catching "what is going around?"

- Is your blood sugar steady?

- Are you having carb cravings or crashes?

General Guidelines

- Eat as many fiber-rich, nonstarchy vegetables as you would like.

- Base your starchy carbohydrate intake on your activity level and your individual body type. If you are very active eat two to three handfuls of starchy carbs per day (yams, root vegetables, fruits, gluten-free grains, sweet potatoes, etc.) If you are less active aim for half that amount.

- Eat one handful of starchy carbs (listed above) in the meal following your workout. If your goal is fat loss this may be the only starchy carbs you eat in a day.

NOTE: *A handful is roughly half a cup.*

- Eat as few as possible refined, sugary carbs. Leave these carbs for special occasions, such as dessert at a fancy restaurant or a slice of cake on your birthday. Then eat them slowly. *Even then, opt for a gluten-free or grain-free homemade version.*

- Always eat slowly and to 80 percent full.

- Stay active. Combine regular exercise with lots of low-intensity daily movement.

Remember, if you adjust your carbohydrate intake, you will likely have to rebalance your plate. Carbs don't work alone; protein, fiber, and fat intake may need to be adjusted as well. For example, instead of spaghetti have spaghetti squash with olive oil drizzled on top. If we feed our bodies with the right balance of protein, carbs, and healthy fats, then our bodies get used to the slow burn of fuel.

 ## TIPS

- Eliminate "sneaky" sugars, like sweetened sauces or nut butters.

- Drink water instead of juice. Flavor water with lemon, lime, orange, or cucumber.

- Eat a half of yam with ghee instead of processed sugary carbs.

- Make a minimally sweetened homemade, whole-food, grain-free muffin, cookie, or pancake.

- Identify a regular occurring "carb craving situation" and find a substitute. At 3 p.m. have an apple with nut butter instead of heading for the vending machine.

Eat the right types of carbs, in the right amounts, consistently. Work to be a little bit better with your choices each week.

PERSONALIZE YOUR CARB INTAKE

You will need to modify your carb intake gradually by making small changes in order to identify your **carbohydrate tolerance/tipping point**. This is the amount of carbohydrates that is low enough to initiate fat loss (*if that is your goal*), but high enough to maintain energy, reduce cravings, and keep hunger at bay. Remember, lower is not always better when it comes to carbohydrates.

Ways to personalize your carbohydrate intake are:

- **Eat for the season.** In the summer, maybe you increase your fruit intake because it is in season and you are more active.

- **Test blood sugar.** It was critical for us to figure out how many carbs we can tolerate.

- **Eat for activity/exercise level.** On the days you are more active, increase your carbs. On the days you are less active, don't eat as many. Aim to eat your starchy carbs in the meal after your workout.

- **Hunger, energy, and cravings can help you to zero in to your carb tolerance.** Start with around a hundred grams per day, and then pay attention to fat-loss results while monitoring hunger, energy, and cravings. *A hundred grams of carbs is roughly six to eight servings of nonstarchy vegetables, one to two servings of fruit, and one-half to one medium-size yam.*[20]

- **Pay attention to mood, motivation, digestion, focus, and sleep.** Proper carbohydrate response should be no

20   Jade Teta, "The Carbohydrate Tipping Point," *Metabolic Effect* (blog), June 14, 2010, www.metaboliceffect.com/the-carbohydrate-tipping-point/.

hunger between meals, no cravings, and increased energy. You should feel motivated and focused without anxiety or depression. Gas and bloating should be minimal or nonexistent and sleep should normalize.

Figuring out your personal carbohydrate tolerance/tipping point can be challenging and frustrating. If you are sticking to the previous *General Guidelines*, you are moving in the right direction. Don't be afraid to make small changes for a couple weeks and see what happens. Notice how your body looks and feels when you make these changes. If you have been "low carb" for some time, try eating more healthy, high-fiber, unprocessed carbs on the days when you are more active or training hard.

CARBOHYDRATES AND ACTIVITY

Activity affects how your body uses the carbohydrates that you eat. The more active you are, the more carbs you will use for fuel rather than being stored as fat. And the opposite is true, the less active you are, the more you will store carbs as fat rather than fuel.

If you want to improve your body's response to carbohydrates, become more active! Activity tells our bodies to send the carbs we eat to the right place: our muscles, liver, and brains, rather than our fat cells. The good news is the more you move, the better the carbohydrate system works. Exercise and daily movement helps our bodies use carbs effectively. Keep in mind, carbohydrates are a fuel source; help them do their job by eating moderate amounts and staying active.

chapter 9

THE TRUTH ABOUT CARBOHYDRATES

All carbs are not bad, and all carbs are not the same.

Let's clear up *carb confusion*. Carbohydrates are large groups of organic compounds occurring in foods and living tissues. They include sugars, starch, and cellulose. Carbohydrates contain hydrogen and oxygen in the same ratio as water and can typically be broken down to release energy in the body. They are one of three main macronutrients, along with protein and fat.

Since carbohydrates are a big group of molecules, you can imagine them as chains made up of links. The links are rings of simple sugars. Smaller chains with fewer links are known as sugars or saccharides. Call these *simple carbohydrates* (honey, maple syrup, candy, soft drinks). Longer chains with more links are known as starches or polysaccharides. Call these *complex carbohydrates* (green vegetables, starchy vegetables, beans).

When we digest carbohydrates, enzymes in our GI tract break down the carbohydrate chain by snapping off the links. Because of their structure, some carbohydrates digest more slowly than others. Slower digesting carbs tend to be starchier (rather than sweeter) and more fibrous. These carbs keep our appetite, energy, and blood sugar more level and help to keep us more satisfied. *All of which is good!*

How carbohydrates act in our bodies largely depends on their chain structure and the allergy-producing potential of the carb. The longer and more complex the chain, the slower it digests, if it breaks down at all. The shorter the chain, the faster our bodies will digest and absorb it. This is why simpler carbs tend to give us blood-sugar highs. Simple sugars are fast tracked into our bloodstream.

Insulin is then secreted to get nutrients into the cells as quickly as possible. More complex carbs break down much more slowly. Your insulin doesn't panic, and you feel a constant, steady energy level. *All carbs are not created equal!* A gram of pure glucose or fructose does not act the same as a gram of lactose or a gram of pectin. To our bodies, a processed granola bar is not the same as a stalk of celery.

Choose complex, high-fiber carbs (non-starchy vegetables) for most of your meals. These carbs will help regulate blood sugar, feed gut bacteria, and provide fiber, all of which keeps our bodies functioning optimally.

To achieve and maintain weight loss, eat carbs with the highest fiber relative to sugar/starch in unlimited amounts. Think non-starchy vegetables. Starchy and sweet carbs like yams, sweet potatoes, plantains, beans, and rice must be managed more closely. Vegetables and fruit (the less sweet ones) may have less fiber than whole grains and beans, but they have far less starch/sugar, a much higher water content, and are non-allergy-producing.

In regard to food sensitivities, *all grains and beans* are usually avoided because of their concentration of gluten, lectins, and saponins, which can create negative effects for the immune system and fat loss. It is important to complete an elimination/detox program to identify if grains and beans work in your body. Allergy/sensitivity-free carbs include yams, plantains, root vegetables, sweet potatoes, etc.

BE SMART ABOUT YOUR CARBS

Think of carbohydrates as being on a continuum from *better* (high fiber, more nourishing, health promoting) to *less optimal* (low fiber, less nourishing, health harming). Some choices are simply better than others. Instead of labeling carbs as *good or bad,* ask yourself some of these questions:

- How can I move along the carb continuum toward higher quality carbohydrate choices?

- How can I add value to my supportive nutrition plan and my body?

- How can I make just one small change today to be just a little better with my carb choices?

What Are Smart Carbs?

Smart carbs give us the good stuff that our bodies need, want, and can use in the right ways. This includes nutrients such as vitamins, minerals, antioxidants, other phytonutrients, fiber, and water. They provide our body with sustained slow-burning energy. These types of carbs are health promoting, slow digesting, and nutrient rich.

High-Fiber Carbs

These include most vegetables, most fruits, legumes, beans, and lentils. These carbs digest slowly and keep you feeling full and energized for a long time. They are rich in vitamins, minerals, and phytonutrients, and good for you. Note: Some people cannot tolerate legumes, beans, and lentils due to a variety of reasons. These foods can stimulate a negative inflammatory reaction in the body.

Starchy Carbs

These include sweet/starchy carbs such as: bananas, plantain, fresh figs/dates, starchy tubers (potatoes, sweet potatoes, taro, yuca), whole grain rice, quinoa, and corn. Like high-fiber carbs, these foods are also usually higher in fiber and beneficial nutrients. They also digest fairly slowly. Most of these foods are *healthier*, but they are more carbohydrate dense than high-fiber carbs. *Pay close attention to how you feel, as some people cannot tolerate many of these carbohydrates due to blood sugar imbalances.*

For example, it would take about six and a half cups of broccoli to match the carb content in one cup of quinoa.

Not So SMART Carbs

These foods include pastries, cakes, cupcakes, muffins, cookies, candy, milk chocolate, fruit juices, soda, bars (including most protein and nutrition bars), other sweetened drinks (sports drinks, coffee drinks, etc.), dried fruit, raisins, dried cranberries, banana chips, and pretty much anything that is processed and/or comes frozen or in a box. *The only exception to this may be minimally sweetened, homemade, whole-food, grain-free baked goods.*

These refined carbs have almost no fiber or beneficial nutrients, they actually subtract value from our bodies. They digest and absorb quickly, which leads to a blood sugar rush followed by a crash, insulin spikes, and, potentially, rebound eating because of the blood sugar roller coaster. These foods don't fill you up, leave you satisfied, or provide you with nourishment. *They just make you feel lousy in the end and leave you wanting more!*

NOTE: *Keep it simple.*

More fiber and nutrients + whole foods = MORE VALUE

Less fiber and fewer nutrients + processing = LESS VALUE

FRUIT

Fruits contain a mix of carbohydrate types, such as simple sugars, starches, and soluble and insoluble fiber. Simple sugars break down quickly in the body, while fiber slows digestion. Fruit has a small amount of fructose plus some other slower digesting carbohydrates types, vitamins, minerals, phytonutrients, and fiber. It gives you sustained energy and lots of other good stuff.

Our bodies know what to do with fresh, whole, unprocessed fruits. When we eat fresh fruit slowly, mindfully, in moderation, we generally feel satisfied and our sugar cravings diminish.

Keep in Mind

- **Eat fruit according to your activity level.** On the days that we train or are moving more in general, we will eat more fruit because our bodies can handle it better. If we have a day when we do yoga and are sitting the majority of the day, we will typically have one serving of fruit or not have it at all.

- **Eat a 3:1 ratio of vegetables to fruit.** Focus on getting in seven to nine servings of vegetables per day and then fill in with fruit. It can be too easy to do the opposite.

- **Avoid high-fructose corn syrup and other forms of fructose.** Choose fresh foods instead of processed versions.

Ask yourself...

- How does fruit work for my body?

- Does fruit fill me up and make me feel satisfied?

- Does fruit satisfy my sugar cravings, or make you crave more sugar?

- Do you digest fruit well, or do you find yourself a bit "off" after some kinds of fruit?

- Do you feel good and have lots of energy when you eat fruit (or certain types of fruit)?

Experiencing Discomfort

Real life is full of obstacles and challenges. If you are used to using carbohydrates as a coping mechanism, it can be hard to cut down on sugary and starchy foods when life stress presents itself. It's normal to want comfort and security. When we seek out high-carb foods, we are really seeking a feeling, a feeling of connection, security, happiness, and pleasure. It is very important to recognize that food can be a drug.

Next time a comfort food craving hits ask yourself:

- What do I want to feel?

- How am I expecting this food to change my mood?

- What is the "hit" that I think this food will give me?

Pause and think about the outcome you really want.

 ## COPING WITHOUT FOOD

Reaching for carbohydrates and sugar when Janell experienced stress was something she struggled with for the better part of her life. The three things that have made the biggest difference for her in not fighting this battle anymore have been:

- Practicing mindfulness and being present.

- Identifying that eating *x* food is not going to change the situation; it is only going to make her feel worse in the long run.

- Having healthier options to turn to when she "just needs something" or wants comfort food, her go-tos are 85 percent dark chocolate, coconut butter, grain-free pizza, and herbal tea.

Managing stress without food really goes back to your self-care toolbox. *What else can you do when a comfort food craving hits?* Identifying what will work for you is crucial in managing "emotional eating."

When a comfort craving hits, Janell will:

- Pet her dog.

- Get outside for ten minutes for some fresh air.

- ▫ Have a cup of herbal tea.

- ▫ Call a friend.

- ▫ Take five minutes to just breathe.

- ▫ Take a hot bath or shower.

- ▫ Journal.

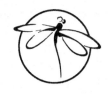

chapter 10

UNDERSTANDING SUGAR

Sugar is detrimental to your health, well-being, and weight-loss goals.

Sugar is *very* addicting, as well as comforting. We all have had a craving that nothing else other than sugar can satisfy. There is a reason for that: we need sugar to live. In fact, our brains demand a constant supply of glucose to function: if we weren't drawn to sugar, we simply wouldn't survive. However, there is such a thing as too much sugar, and nearly *everyone* in our country is eating too much.

It's easy to do—sugar is hiding in 75 percent of the six hundred thousand items you can buy in grocery stores. Some sugary items are pretty obvious, but others might surprise you. It hides in tomato sauce; salad dressings; sauces; chicken, vegetable, or beef broth; nut butters; pasta sauces; deli meats; and even baby food!

In a video that went viral on YouTube,[21] Dr. Robert Lustig (a pediatric endocrinologist) explained in layperson's terms just how dangerous sugar is for us. He argued that the current obesity epidemic is due to the marked increase in people's consumption of fructose over the last thirty years. Dr. Lustig points out that fructose is toxic in large quantities because it is metabolized in the liver in the same way as alcohol, which drives fat storage and makes the brain think it is hungry.

> *To watch Dr. Lustig's compelling video on YouTube, search for "Sugar: the Bitter Truth" or enter the following URL: https://www.youtube.com/watch?v=dBnniua6-oM.*

THE NEGATIVE IMPACT OF SUGAR

Sugar is one of the top offenders in our current epidemic of high cholesterol, obesity, type 2 diabetes, high blood pressure, insulin resistance, and metabolic syndrome. The problem is that people are consuming much more sugar than their body needs and much more than their body can metabolize.

One part of your body that sugar is affecting is your brain. New research is showing that your sweet tooth is leading to the literal decay of your brain. Diabetics are more likely to get dementia, but now it appears that when a person's blood sugar levels get to the high end of the normal range, important areas in the brain begin to

---

21   Robert Lustig, "Sugar: The Bitter Truth," *University of California Television*, www.youtube.com/watch?v=dBnniua6-oM

shrink. These areas are the hippocampus and the amygdala—areas that are key players in memory and mental skills.[22]

There is also evidence that sugar directly affects our immune response, weakening our ability to fight off infection. In fact, "eating or drinking 100 grams (8 TBSP) of sugar, the equivalent of 2.5 12-ounce cans of soda, can reduce the ability of white blood cells to kill germs by 40 percent. The immune-suppressing effect of sugar starts less than thirty minutes after ingestion and may last for five hours."[23]

Our mood is also impacted by sugar. When you eat a lot of sugar, you are going to have abrupt peaks and drops in your blood sugar levels, which will manifest themselves in various ways. You may find that you are tired, irritable, and depressed, and you may even have crying spells.

 ## A RECIPE FOR FIGHTS

About six years ago, before we were as committed to a whole food, nutrient-dense diet, we were driving home from visiting Janell's family in Wisconsin and decided to stop at a new Dunkin' Donuts that had opened. Growing up in Wisconsin, Janell had never had Dunkin' Donuts before so we decided to get some so she could try them. I hadn't had them in years so it was special for me, as well.

22   David Perlmutter and Kristen Loberg, *Grain Brain* (Boston: Little, Brown and Company, 2013), 122.
23   Bill Sears, "Harmful Effects of Excess Sugar," *AskDrSears* (bog), www.askdrsears. com/topics/family-nutrition/sugar/harmful-effects-excess-sugar

When we stopped for these donuts, we were about three and a half hours from home. Soon after, we got into a heated fight! About what? Neither of us remembers! We actually enjoy our roads trips, so for us to be in an intense fight was unprecedented.

We were nearly home when we stopped for a minute and recognized exactly what had just happened— sugar at its finest. It was a complete blood sugar spike and then crash, which resulted in altering our moods, this time to complete anger. On the positive side, we were able to pinpoint what had happened and forgive each other for anything that was said during our sugar rage!

—Justin

Pause for a moment and think about how many times you snap at people around you. Could it be the sugar talking? Do you feel as though you can't control your moods and emotions? Do you find yourself feeling depressed or low?

In fact, studies have shown that those who eat a lot of processed foods (which are loaded with refined sugar and refined carbs) were at a 58 percent higher risk for depression than those who ate a diet higher in whole, unprocessed foods.

HOW SUGAR IS PROCESSED IN OUR BODIES?

In today's Standard American Diet, fructose is the sugar of choice. It's not that fructose itself is bad (fruit contains fructose), but it is the huge quantities in which it is consumed that is the issue.

The two main reasons that fructose is so damaging to your body are: your body metabolizes fructose in a much different way from glucose, and the large quantities in which fructose is consumed makes the negative effects that much more damaging.

The burden of processing fructose falls solely on your liver. Your liver only breaks down about 20 percent of glucose, and since nearly every cell in your body uses glucose, it is normally "burned up" after consumption.

So where does all the fructose go once you consume it? You guessed it, right to your thighs—it is turned into fat!

The problem is our bodies are simply not designed to carry the load of fructose that nearly everyone in our country consumes. When fructose is separated from the fiber in which it naturally occurs, the result can be deadly. Even fruit juice is harmful. *Your body cannot tell the difference between fructose from a glass of orange juice and fructose from a can of Mountain Dew.*

What About Fruit?

Fruit also contain fructose, but whole fruits also contain vitamins and other beneficial antioxidants that reduce the hazardous effects of fructose. Juice, on the other hand, is a different story and is as damaging as soda. A glass of juice is full of fructose and lacks the antioxidants and fiber of whole fruit. We need to just be mindful of our fruit consumption and match it with our activity level and health and fitness goals.

TYPES OF SUGAR

All sugars are *not* created equal. But all sugar can negatively impact our health and weight-loss results.

Here is a basic overview of popular sugars and sweeteners:

- Dextrose, fructose, and glucose are all monosaccharides, known as simple sugars. The primary difference between them is how your body metabolizes them. Glucose and dextrose are essentially the same sugar. However, food manufacturers usually use dextrose in their ingredient list.

- Simple sugars can combine to form more complex sugars, like the disaccharide sucrose (table sugar), which is half glucose and half fructose. High-fructose corn syrup is 55 percent fructose and 45 percent glucose.

- Ethanol (drinking alcohol) is not a sugar, although beer and wine contain residual sugars and starches in addition to alcohol.

- Sugar alcohols like xylitol, glycerol, sorbitol, maltitol, mannitol, and erythritol are neither sugars nor alcohols but are becoming increasingly more popular. They are absorbed from your intestine; therefore, they provide fewer calories than sugar but often cause bloating, diarrhea, and gas.

- Sucralose (Splenda) is not a sugar but instead a chlorinated artificial sweetener in line with aspartame and saccharin and can result in negative health consequences.

- Agave syrup is highly processed and is usually 80 percent fructose.

- Honey is about 53 percent fructose but is completely natural in its raw form and can have many health benefits when used in moderation.

- Stevia is a highly sweet herb, which is safe in its natural form. The problem is that food manufacturers use fillers in many stevia products. Opt for a natural brand such as NuNaturals or Sweet Leaf.[24]

There are approximately fifty-six different names used for sugar. Be sure to read food labels, as sugar can be the single largest ingredient but listed in various names within the ingredient list.

HOW DO WE INCORPORATE SUGAR INTO OUR LIVES?

When it comes to sweeteners, the most important thing we have learned is that once your palate changes, you need *much less* than previously. You may have also experienced this. You eat something that you used to really enjoy, and now you think, "*That's too sweet.*" Honestly, it can be somewhat disappointing.

Once you have abstained from sugar and sweeteners for any given period of time, you notice that your taste receptors for sweet have changed. Carrots, butternut squash, 85 percent dark chocolate, and fruit taste really sweet!

When we say that to people, often they give us some weird looks, but some of you know exactly what we are talking about! Giving your body a complete break from sugar for a given time is a really good idea because it is almost inevitable that it will creep back in, one way or another, in some capacity.

All sugars and sweeteners, whether they contain calories or not, can contribute to weight gain and/or prevent weight loss.

We have previously addressed how all calories are not created equal and that the most important thing is to eat high-quality, nutri-

---

24   Joseph Mercola, "Fructose: This Addictive Commonly Used Food Feeds Cancer Cells, Triggers Weight Gain, and Promotes Premature Aging," *Mercola.com* (blog), http://articles.mercola.com/sites/articles/archive/2010/04/20/sugar-dangers.aspx

ent-dense food. Several studies have shown that any sweet sensation can cause an insulin release in your body.

Remember that the hormone insulin puts our bodies into a fat storage mode. This is only part of the problem with non-calorie sweeteners. In addition to having negative effects on our metabolism, these sugars and sweeteners are full of chemicals.

Artificial sweeteners are known to cause health issues, such as: migraines/headaches, nausea/vomiting, change in moods, fatigue, diarrhea, joint pain, memory loss, and sleep problems, just to name a few. Those things alone are enough for us to stay away from these factory-made sugars and sweeteners. For your waistline and your health, avoid them *completely*.

Natural sweeteners are a better choice over those that come from a lab or factory. This is true for any food we consume. Real whole foods that come from nature are *always* a better choice than anything made in a lab or factory. Our bodies recognize and know what to do with natural food.

Nonchemical sweeteners include: raw honey, molasses, date sugar, palm sugar, coconut sugar, fruit juice, grade B maple syrup, cane sugar, and green leaf stevia. These sweeteners are not necessarily "*healthy*," nonchemical simply means that they are refined from something that was originally found in nature and are not made from chemicals. Most of the time, these nonchemical sweeteners can be metabolized by your body, while chemical sweeteners cannot and are instead considered toxins within our system. Just like all toxins, they are stored in our fat cells.

Chemical sweeteners include: aspartame (Equal), saccharin, stevia (Truvia and Stevia in the Raw), and sucralose (Splenda).[25]

---

25   Diane Sanfilippo, "The Dish on Sugar & Sweeteners," *balancedbites* (blog), April 12, 2011, http://balancedbites.com/the-dish-on-sugar-sweeteners/

It is always best to limit your consumption of sugars and sweeteners no matter what the source is. It is important to read labels and find *hidden sweeteners*. Sugar and sweeteners are hiding *everywhere,* including places you wouldn't even think of, like chicken broth!

NOTE: *It is also important to check the labels on protein shakes and bars. Oftentimes, they will contain one or more of the chemical sweeteners listed above.*

Always check the sugar grams listed on labels. Then look at the ingredients for any words ending in -ose or -ol. That means it is a form of sugar or a sugar alcohol. Examples include: sucralose, glucose, sucrose, fructose, dextrose, maltose, lactose, mannitol, sorbitol, and xylitol.

Other words to look for are syrup, sugar, nectar, and crystals. Things like *organic brown rice syrup* are still sources of sweetener and you need to be aware of them and minimize exposure. When reading any ingredient list, the first item listed is the most abundant ingredient, and so on down the list. If a sugar or sweetener is listed within the first few ingredients, then the item has a high content of sweetener in comparison to the other ingredients. Food manufacturers have caught on to the fact that consumers are aware of this so they will include three, four, or more different sweeteners in an item. Look for how many different types of sweeteners are in an item; you may be surprised.

It's okay to have nonchemical sweeteners like raw honey and grade B maple syrup in moderation. Ideally, use organic, nonchemical sweeteners whenever possible. *The key is moderation.*

We find that a lot less sweetener is required than most recipes call for. If a recipe calls for half a cup of raw honey, we will typically use a quarter of a cup. If a recipe calls for two tablespoons of honey in addition to fruit, such as mashed banana, we will likely leave out the honey all together.

Keep in mind . . .

- *All* sugars and sweeteners, whether they contain calories or not, can contribute to weight gain or prevent weight loss.

- Sweeteners that come from nature are a better choice over those that come from a lab or factory.

- It is always best to limit your consumption of sugars and sweeteners no matter what the source is.[26]

SUGAR IS A DRUG

Nutrient-poor, high-sugar, salty, carbohydrate-dense foods are addicting and alter our pleasure, reward, and emotional pathways in the brain.

Sugar can sometimes have a calming effect in the moment, but it is an addictive substance. A 2007 study by a team of French researchers showed that sugar could be more rewarding than cocaine! Wheat, which is broken down into sugar in the body, actually binds to the opiate receptors in the brain! Two factors that reinforce and make the addictive properties of sugar-filled, high-carbohydrate foods worse are chronic stress and lack of sleep.

What foods do you "crave" when you are stressed or running on little sleep? Foods rich in carbohydrate, because they will increase serotonin, our *"feel good"* hormone. We then overeat these *"Fran-*

---

26   Mercola, "Fructose."

kenfoods" (*high-sugar, high trans-fat, high-preservative, unnatural, processed foods*) because we never reach satiation due to their lack of nutrients. Eating delicious food with the nutrition and satiety that nature intended is the solution to this problem.

Why Is Sugar So Hard to Stay Away From?

If you have leaky gut, a gastrointestinal infection, parasites, yeast, or the excess bacteria associated with SIBO (*Small Intestinal, Bacterial, Overgrowth*), then your sugar cravings can be more intense. These bugs in your intestines are begging you to feed them so they send sugar-craving signals directly to your brain. The first few days off of sugar can be very difficult and it may even feel like you are going through drug withdrawals, but we promise you that you will feel so much better off of sugar! That may be hard to grasp right now, but after avoiding sugar, you will notice that you no longer have cravings and it isn't as appealing as it once was.

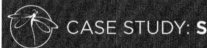 CASE STUDY: **SUGAR HIGH**

I suffered from severe depression for many years. My doctor tried numerous different antidepressants and antipsychotic medications to try to find the right combination to stabilize the depressive symptoms. The medications made me unable to feel anything, and my thought process was very sluggish. My husband and I began doing some research on the brain chemistry with depression. We asked my doctor if I could be weaned off the medication while, at the same time, work with a nutritionist to see if diet could help stabilize my mood and improve the depressive symptoms. What I discovered as I changed my diet was that simple carbohydrates and sugar had a negative effect on my mood. Over a year's time I was weaned off of my medication. Through a diet low in sugar and with regular exercise, I have been able to stay off of antidepressant medication. I have been medication free for six years now, but I need to monitor my food intake pretty closely. If I eat too much sugar or simple carbs I will have mood swings that can be quite severe.

—Theresa Endres

DOES SUGAR FIT INTO A SUPPORTIVE NUTRITION PLAN?

Even though sugar, in particular fructose, is very detrimental to our bodies, we don't think it is realistic to live in a reality where you never eat sugar again. However, through education, preparing your own food, and conscious, mindful eating you can *drastically* cut down on your sugar consumption.

THREE TIPS FOR CUTTING DOWN ON SUGAR

- **Cut sugar out of your diet for *at least* three weeks completely.** Your body can become "sensitized" to sugar and its effects. After you do so, your body will be less reactive to sugar. This will also help you to realize how much sugar you are actually consuming. It is likely *far more* than you realize. It can be VERY beneficial to do several mini resets throughout the year that last anywhere from 3 days to several weeks when you choose to cut out sugar completely to reset your palate, blood sugar, and improve your hormones.

- **Make the vast majority of your own desserts and baked goods.** This way you can control how much sugar you add. You can likely cut the sugar in a recipe in half and it will still be sweet enough for you.

- **Consume natural forms of sugar such as fruit and raw honey, and completely avoid processed packaged foods that contain high-fructose corn syrup, chemicals sweeteners, sugar alcohols, or other forms of sugar.**

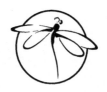

chapter 11

FAT IS YOUR FRIEND

We mentioned earlier that one of the biggest nutrition myths of all time is that dietary fat is bad for our health. Because there is so much confusion about fat, we wanted to include more information and education for you than *"just eat healthy fats at each meal."*

In fact, a review coauthored by Walter Willett, chair of the department of nutrition at the Harvard School of Public Health, stated the following: *"It is now increasingly recognized that the low-fat campaign has been based on little scientific evidence and may have caused unintended health consequences."*[27]

There was a time where we embraced foods that contained natural fat, but somewhere along the line we started to believe that dietary fat equated to body fat. We avoided foods high in saturated fat and cholesterol in hopes that that would prevent disease and improve our health.

---

27   Liz Wolfe, *Eat the Yolks* (Victory Belt Publishing, Inc., 2014), 34.

Avoiding fat isn't the answer and it's not working! The government recommendations for eating a high-carb, low-fat diet is and has been *very* profitable for certain parts of our medical and pharmaceutical industries. Unfortunately, it has not been as kind to many of us or our family and friends.

Despite lower fat diets and being cautious of the cholesterol, people are still sick and suffering with the same diseases that doing so were supposed to prevent. In fact, as a society we've got worse!

WHERE IT ALL STARTED

In the early 1950s, Ancel Keys put together *The Seven Countries Study*, in which it *appeared* that the more fat a country consumed, the more prevalent heart disease was.[28] The reason why this paper was so convincing was that it did in fact show that the more fat a country consumed the higher the rates of heart disease but only because Keys conveniently *threw out* all of the data that proved otherwise!

There were numerous countries that consumed high amounts of fat and showed low rates of cardiovascular disease, while other countries showed high rates of cardiovascular disease and ate little dietary fat. If the entirety of *The Seven Countries Study* was considered, it would have included twenty-two countries, and the conclusion from this larger (and more accurate) set of data would have been, "There is no relationship between fat intake and cardiovascular disease."

The idea that fat was the cause for cardiovascular disease was appealing for people. And because this was post-World War II, the government had a sense of do-goodery. This drove the government

---

28   "Ancel Keys—Launching the Seven Countries Study" The Seven Countries Study, 2016, http://www.sevencountriesstudy.com/about-the-study/investigators/ancel-keys/.

and the McGovern Commission to champion the fat-heart hypothesis. To feed this hypothesis, researchers reasoned that if Americans were fat, and rates of heart disease were higher than other countries, then they should reduce the fat in their diet.

Just because the assumption that fat makes people fat and causes heart disease makes sense, doesn't make it *true*.

THE IMPORTANCE OF FAT

Fat is important for normal cell functioning and nervous system function. Your brain and nerves are made of mostly fat. Fat supports satiety, is necessary for normal hormone production, and is a great long-lasting source of energy.

Fats come in various forms and structures and can be divided into three categories: saturated, monounsaturated, and polyunsaturated. These different types of fat have different physiological roles.

According to Dr. Mary Enig, author of *Know Your Fats*, "Fats and oils (technically called lipids) are basically made up of collections of molecules called triglycerides. If the collection is liquid at ambient temperature, it's called an oil; if it is solid, it's called a fat."

Saturated fats have been given a bad rap. The reality is that saturated fats are usually benign and some are quite helpful. Saturated fats are found in animal fats (eggs, dairy, meats, butter, cheeses, etc.), coconut oil, and red palm oil.

If your intake of saturated fat comes from quality sources and your carbohydrate level comes mostly from nonstarchy vegetables and small amounts of fruit, then you have little to no risk of developing cardiovascular disease. However, a high intake of saturated fats, paired with a high intake of dietary carbohydrate, is a combination for disease and an early grave.

Coconut and coconut oil are some of the most widely popular saturated fats. Coconut oil is made up of medium-chain fatty acids, which yield 25 percent fewer calories per gram than most other fats. The fat in coconut oil is digested and metabolized differently than other fats. In fact, it can even help you to lose weight.

The fats from coconut do not get bundled into lipoproteins, which seek out a fat cell to expand and make fatter. Instead, they go straight to the liver, where they are used for energy. The medium-chain fatty acids found in coconut also help your body blaze through slower-burning, long-chain triglycerides as well. A recent study showed that medium-chain fatty acids given over a six-day period can increase diet-induced fat burning by 50 percent.

Monounsaturated fats are found in olive oil, nuts and nut butters, and avocados. Benefits of monounsaturated fats include improved insulin sensitivity, improved glucagon response, and decreased cholesterol levels. Plant sources of these fats also provide your cell membranes with fat-soluble antioxidants. These antioxidants help to prevent oxidative damage in our bodies.

Monounsaturated fats were the primary fat in our ancestors' diets. If you want to optimize how you look, feel, and perform, it is important to incorporate these fats into your supportive nutrition plan.

Polyunsaturated fats are found in flax seeds, fish and fish oil, grass-fed meats, nuts and nut butters, and vegetable oils. These are known as the essential fats. Essential fats are those that we cannot make and therefore must obtain from our diets. Not getting enough of these fats, or in the right ratios, can lead to *big* problems down the road. Polyunsaturated fats are made up of omega-3 and omega-6 fatty acids.

Omega-3 fats are anti-inflammatory and omega-6 fats are generally pro-inflammatory. Omega-3 fats are made up of alpha-linolenic acid (ALA), eicosapentaenoic acid (EPA), and docosahexaenoic acid (DHA). omega-6 fats are made up of linoleic acid (LA), gamma linolenic acid (GLA), dihomo-gamma-linolenic acid (DGLA), and arachidonic acid (AA).

In addition to increasing inflammation, the polyunsaturated omega-6 linoleic acid found in refined seed oils and trans fats increases the permeability of the intestinal tract (leaky gut).

Refined oils (listed on page 64) will also skew your dietary ratio of omega-6 to omega-3 fats in the wrong direction. A high dietary ratio of omega-6 to omega-3 is associated with more inflammation. It is estimated that the SAD has *fifteen to twenty times* as many omega-6 to omega-3; the ideal ratio should be close to 1:1. *This is the problem with fat intake.* Our bodies are designed for roughly equal amounts of pro- and anti-inflammatory fats in our diets.

This high ratio can contribute to accelerated aging and the development of many chronic diseases: cardiovascular disease, cancer, arthritis, and other inflammatory and autoimmune conditions. Polyunsaturated fats include both omega-6 and omega-3 fats, which are both essential to your health but have a very high oxidative potential. Too much polyunsaturated fat can be detrimental to your health.

Nuts and seeds may also be problematic, as they tend to have higher omega-6 fatty acids, which can drive up your dietary fatty acid ratios toward a pro-inflammation (omega-6) state. Use nuts and seeds as you would a condiment instead of as daily snacks.

To improve your health and reduce inflammation, decrease your total polyunsaturated fat intake and improve your omega-6 to omega-3 ratio by avoiding the listed refined oils. The two most effective ways to do this are by reducing how often you eat out at restaurants (seed oils are almost always used for cooking) and avoiding packaged and processed foods.

Trans fats are only about fifty years old and our bodies and metabolism have *no idea* what to do with them. Trans fats are made when polyunsaturated fats from corn, soybean, and similar oils are exposed to heat, hydrogen gas, and a catalyst. Anything that is hydrogenated or partially hydrogenated is a trans fat, such as Crisco.

Trans fats are hard on the liver, ruin insulin sensitivity, and wreak havoc on blood lipids. Consume trans fats and high-fructose corn syrup and you will dig yourself an early grave. The good news is that trans fats should become less and less of a problem as they are being removed from restaurants and prepared foods.

BUSTING THE MYTHS ABOUT FAT

The following are the *five biggest myths* about dietary fat and cholesterol.

Myth #1: Fat Makes You Fat

Let's cover this right off the bat: the increase in obesity in America happened right about the time fat and cholesterol were made out to be the bad guy. **Through decades of low-fat diets and fat-free processed foods we, as a country, have just gotten heavier.**

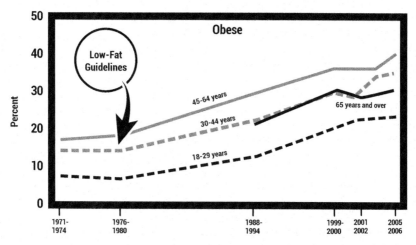

Obesity rates took off after low-fat guidelines were established.

Source: *National Center for Health Statistics (US), Health, United States, 2008: With Special Feature on the Health of Young Adults (Hyattsville, MD: National Center for Health Statistics (US), 2009).*

The fact remains that we *need* fat in our diets. Dietary fat helps your body utilize fat-soluble vitamins. Eating fat with each meal also helps to stabilize your appetite by affecting satiety hormones, keeping you full for longer periods of time. Fat provides your body with consistent energy by not triggering an insulin release, as do sugar and processed carbohydrates.

The rationale behind dietary fat making people fat was that fat has more calories (*nine calories/gram*) than protein and carbohydrate (*four calories/gram*). So if you consume more calories than you burn, you will gain weight. Therefore, reduce fat and the chance of consuming too many calories will also be reduced. This idea makes sense, so much so that no one bothered to actually make sure it was *true*. No one thought about the fact that carbohydrate, and the insulin it releases, actually drives hunger and fat storage.

The fact that protein and fat intake provide satiation, reducing overall calorie intake was also overlooked.

143

Myth #2: A Low-Fat, High-Carbohydrate Diet Is Optimal

There is no evidence that low-fat diets have any benefits. They do not cause permanent weight loss or reduce the risk of chronic diseases in the long term.

Despite fat having more calories per gram than carbohydrate or protein, studies show that high-fat (and low-carbohydrate) diets actually lead to more weight loss than do low-fat diets. This is because a diet based on whole, real, unprocessed foods allows us to control and manage our hormones, cravings, and hunger—which leads to weight loss.

The key is to eat protein, vegetables, healthy fats, fruit, and the right amount of starchy carbohydrates to fuel activity levels in order to keep our blood sugar and insulin level in check.

On the flip side, a low-fat diet leaves us feeling unsatisfied, which can lead to overeating. Low fat also typically means higher in processed starchy carbohydrates causing a higher blood sugar and, therefore, a stronger insulin response potentially leading to increased fat storage.

When we started eating "low-fat" in America, we gained weight because our diets were much higher in processed carbohydrates and sugar.

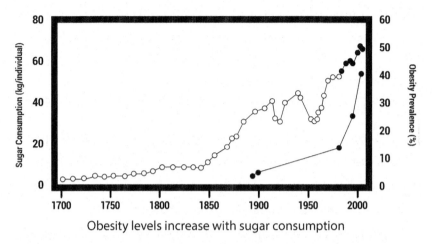

Obesity levels increase with sugar consumption

Source: *RJ Johnson et al., 2007, "Potential Role of Sugar (Fructose) in the Epidemic of Hypertension, Obesity, and the Metabolic Syndrome, Diabetes, Kidney Disease, and Cardiovascular Disease," The American Journal of Clinical Nutrition 86(4): 899–906.*

If you take the fat out of food, you must add something to make it taste good—hello, sugar! The food manufactures caught on to this very quickly, and we were all lead to believe that low-fat crackers, cookies, yogurt, etc., were health foods.

Where did that get us?

Myth #3: Cholesterol-Rich Foods Are Bad

Your body only absorbs 15 percent of the cholesterol you eat. The other 85 percent is excreted. Therefore, the cholesterol you consume has little to do with the cholesterol levels in your bloodstream.

"When we eat more cholesterol, the body produces less," says nutritionist and physician Natasha Campbell-McBride.

Cholesterol is a waxy substance that is an important constituent of cell membranes. The vast majority of cholesterol in the body is made in the liver, while the rest is absorbed from the diet. Cholesterol is the basic raw material that your body uses to make vitamin

D, sex hormones, and bile acids needed for digestion. Therefore, we do not need to avoid egg yolks, because they are high in cholesterol.[29]

Myth #4: Saturated Fat Increases Risk for Heart Disease

Despite decades of anti-fat propaganda, saturated fat has never been proven to cause heart disease. In fact, saturated fat improves some of its important risk factors. Doctors, media, and those making nutritional recommendations to the public have wrongfully demonized saturated fat.

Saturated fat raises the more favorable "good" (HDL) cholesterol, which are big, fluffy pattern A particles. They tend to change the pattern of your "bad" (LDL) cholesterol, which are small pattern B particles that stick to artery walls and promote atherosclerosis. Several recent studies have shown that greater saturated fat intake is associated with less progression of coronary atherosclerosis, whereas carbohydrate intake is associated with greater progression.

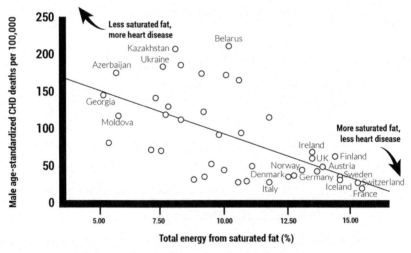

Fig. 1 Saturated fat intake and CHD mortality in Europe (1998)

Source: *R. Hoenselaar, 2012, "Further Response from Hoenselaar," British Journal of Nutrition, 108(5): 939–942.*

---

29 Wolfe, 51–55.

There is no evidence that supports a direct relationship between saturated fat and heart disease. Remember, correlation is not causation.

Myth #5: Seed Oils Are Healthy

Unrefined, natural fat that comes from properly raised animals is not the problem. Rather, the issue is in refined seed oils. Seed and vegetable oils are unhealthy, loaded with omega-6 fatty acids and trans fats that can contribute to disease.

The high doses of omega-6 fatty acids consumed in the SAD increase inflammation in the body. Increased inflammation is the root of all chronic disease.

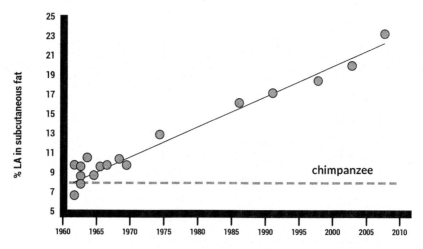

Linoleic Acid in US Body Fat, 1961-2008

Source: Stephan Guyenet, "Seed Oils and Body Fatness—A Problematic Revisit," Whole Health Source (blog), August 21, 2011, http://wholehealth-source.blogspot.com/2011/08/seed-oils-and-body-fatness-problematic.html.

Refined seeds oils also become oxidized because they do not remain stable under light or heat. When we consume these oxidized oils, they get into our cells and can accelerate aging and promote chronic disease, such as cancer and heart disease.

The refinement process that these oils go through strips away any nutrients that may have been there in the first place. The oils from corn, soy, cotton, and canola crops are extracted through a chemical-filled/high-heat process. One of the first steps to increase your health is to avoid refined seed oils as much as possible.[30]

WRAPPING IT UP

Natural fats that occur in properly raised animals, avocados, nuts and seeds, coconut, and olive oil are a part of a healthy supportive nutrition plan. Remember, fat is not the problem. It's the wrong types of fats coming from refined seed oils and trans fats in processed foods that are the problem.

Ideally, you would have an omega-3 to omega-6 ratio, minimally of 1:3 by eating grass-fed meats, wild-caught fish, and limiting your intake of omega-6 fats. Balancing your intake of essential fats will help you to lose fat, gain muscle, increase energy, and look, feel, and perform better!

Superfoods that contain omega-3 fats includes:

- wild Alaskan salmon

- sardines

- anchovies

- mackerel

- herring

- trout

- grass-fed meat

- free-range eggs

---

30   Wolfe, 65–69.

Include fat at each meal to help keep you full and satisfied longer. When you have appropriate amounts of fat in your diet, you actually end up eating fewer total calories because your body has the nutrition that it requires and your taste buds are satisfied.

chapter 12

LIQUIDS

In order to achieve your weight loss goals and improve your health, you will need to pay attention to your liquid calories. Make it a habit to not drink beverages with more than zero calories. *This doesn't mean that diet drinks or sodas that contain artificial sweeteners are a good choice.* Remember, your body doesn't know how to process these artificial sweeteners, nor do we truly understand how they are impacting the human body.

This means removing alcohol, soda (even diet), coffee drinks or lattes, milk (see exception below), fruit juices, energy drinks, and sports drinks. Those morning lattes full of sugar and chemicals can really set you back from achieving your goals. These drinks contain extra sugar that your body doesn't need, are not satiating, and do not contain much, if any, nutrition.

Eat your fruits and vegetables, and drink water as your beverage. Fruit juice has little nutritional value and it will increase blood sugar much more quickly than eating a piece of fruit.

The exception to this would be continuing to incorporate protein shakes into your supportive nutrition plan. Protein shakes can be a way for you to get in some good nutrition when you are on the run and they can be great pre- or post-workout.

NOTE: *We would encourage you to either make your protein shake with water or an unsweetened milk alternative, like almond milk. It is best to make homemade almond milk. If you are going to buy it from the grocery store, buy a brand with a shorter ingredient list and one that does not contain Carrageenan.*

This does not mean that you can *never* drink alcohol or have an almond milk latte every once in a while. What it means is that for a period of time it is important to remove all the beverages listed to understand if they are having a negative impact on your weight and/ or your health.

WATER

It is ideal to drink half your body weight in ounces of water each day. Your body is made up of 60 percent water, and water is absolutely essential for a variety of physiological functions. Your health, performance, and body composition will suffer if you don't drink enough water. Drinking an adequate amount of water each day can aid your digestion. For more optimal digestion, drink water between meals rather than with your meals.

Hydrating first thing in the morning with twelve to twenty ounces of warm water with one tablespoon of pure lemon juice (not from concentrate) can be a great way to increase water consumption for the day. This also can aid in digestion and detoxification, increase your vitamin C intake for the day, and may help you to lose weight.

COFFEE & TEA

Many people don't actually like the taste of *coffee*. What they do like is the taste of a liquid dessert that can pack more than thirty grams of sugar in a small latte. Just think how much sugar is in a large! If you truly enjoy the taste of coffee and you find that it works for your body, then try enjoying it black. Focus on quality: coffee from the gas station will taste *very* different than coffee from a local coffee shop that uses high-quality beans.

Many people have a hard time metabolizing coffee and it leaves them feeling jittery and with low blood sugar symptoms. Notice if an hour or two after you drink coffee you are having carbohydrate cravings or wanting sugar. If this is the case, then it is likely that your body does not metabolize the caffeine in coffee well, and you will want to consider not drinking it or drinking decaf.

Just like alcohol, it is important to go a period of time (at least three weeks) without coffee so that you can truly know how it is affecting you. Coffee often masks poor sleep, drops in energy, or fatigue from improper nutrition or meal timing. You might surprise yourself, as you may feel better and have more energy without coffee! A great coffee alternative is Dandy Blend, a roasted dandelion root with a rich flavor.

Green, black, and herbal teas are also great options. Tea contains much less caffeine than coffee, so most people can tolerate it really well. Tea contains polyphenols and antioxidants that are beneficial to the body. Drinking tea can benefit the body by boosting your immune system, improving your insulin sensitivity, and lowering your cortisol levels.

As with anything else, quality matters. Opt for an organic tea and that comes in quality tea bags, not ones that are bleached or dyed.

ALCOHOL

Alcohol is a toxin to the body and once it enters your bloodstream it starts a chain reaction that will inhibit your metabolism. Many metabolic functions will come to a halt when alcohol is present in your body, including fat burning! Alcohol will also severely dehydrate your body, which can be very harmful to your health and fat loss results. It's not only the alcohol that has a negative impact but also the choices you make after a few drinks. It is not very likely that you will stop eating the nachos when you have had enough or pass up dessert after a few drinks.

Both Janell and I are nondrinkers now, but that wasn't always the case. And we will both tell you that it was much harder to lose weight when alcohol was part of our life. We were not people who could work out and follow a supportive nutrition plan during the week and then drink on the weekends and see results. It just doesn't work that way for most people.

Again, we believe that it is important that you *completely* remove alcohol for a few weeks so that you can understand how it is impacting your ability to lose weight as well as your overall physical, mental, and emotional health. It is also important to understand how you are using alcohol in your life. Only after a period of time without it can you determine how you want it to fit into your overall supportive nutrition plan.

Can you go without alcoholic beverages for three weeks without feeling uncomfortable?

If not, then you may not be using alcohol in moderate amounts. You may be using it to cope with your life.

You may want to ask yourself:

- What am I using alcohol for?

- Why do I feel uncomfortable *not* drinking?

- How often do I drink, how much, around who, and in what situations?

These questions may be difficult to answer, and that is okay. We are not here to judge you. Rather, we want you to become aware if alcohol is more of an issue than you thought it was.

Be honest with yourself, why are you drinking alcohol:

- Do you truly enjoy it?

- Are you drinking because everyone else is and you don't want to be left out?

- Are you drinking to cope with stress or negative emotions?

chapter 13

NUTRITION ON THE GO

PRE/POST-WORKOUT NUTRITION

Pre- and post-workout nutrition are important because you want to be properly fueled for your workout. It may be hard for you to see improvements in your workouts and for you to increase the intensity of your workouts if you are not properly fueled by the food you eat around the time of your workouts.

What you eat before and after a workout will depend on the type of workout you are doing and your individual goals. The information below is geared toward a person who is strength training and has fat-loss goals.

Pre-Workout

This is going to vary based on when you work out and what your body can handle. It is okay to fast before a workout if you feel good during your workouts and your workouts continue to get better.

If you do need to eat before your workout, focus on protein and possibly a little fat, but avoid lots of fruit or carb-dense vegetables.

A carbohydrate-rich meal will increase insulin, putting your body into a fat-storing mode. Examples of a pre-workout "snack" would be: two hard-boiled eggs, some turkey or chicken, or a few strips of homemade beef jerky (without added sugar). An easy go-to for pre-workout can be a high-quality protein shake. Mix a high-quality protein powder with water or unsweetened almond milk, and drink it on the way to your workout. Avoid adding any fruit pre-workout, stick to just protein.

 ## JANELL'S PRE-WORKOUT MEAL

Janell typically works out around 11 a.m., so her pre-workout meal is breakfast, since she eats breakfast around 8 a.m. She aims to have protein, nonstarchy vegetables, and a small amount of fat (whatever is in the protein or what she cooked the vegetables with). An example may be four ounces of a turkey sausage breakfast patty, one cup of steamed green beans, and half a cup of roasted butternut squash.

Post-Workout

Eat within thirty to sixty minutes of your workouts. Have one serving of protein, one to two servings of nonstarchy vegetables, and one serving of starchy carbohydrate. Fruit is *not* your best option here. Examples of a post-workout meal include chicken breast, one cup nonstarchy vegetable, half a cup cooked sweet potato or salmon, one cup nonstarchy vegetable, and half a cup cooked yam.

Your post-workout meal could be a protein shake using high-quality protein powder. An example of a post-workout protein shake would be:

- one cup unsweetened almond milk

- one to two big handfuls of spinach or kale

- one serving of protein powder

- one serving of fruit

SUPPLEMENTS ARE NOT SOLUTIONS

Let's be clear right up front: there is a place for supplements in a supportive nutrition program; however, supplements are *not* solutions. That means you can't just take a pill, powder, or potion and expect to magically get results. They don't solve your weight-loss problem.

Supplements are meant to support nutrition program. And, yes, even if you follow the nutrition plan outlined in this book, you will still lack some nutrients your body needs to function optimally, so you will benefit from some supplements.

If you hear the phrase "nutrient deficiency pandemic," what part of the world would you imagine would be at risk? Third-world countries likely come to mind. You would be partially right, but this pandemic is real and it is global—no nation is exempt.

You may be wondering how the most developed and prosperous country on the earth could have a pandemic of nutrient deficiency. After all, we nearly have more food than we know what to do with. The answer has to do with the *quality* of the food that we are eating. Most Americans eat the Standard American Diet, which ironically is known as the SAD. This diet is high in unhealthy fats and refined sugar and flour, while low in complex carbohydrates, vegetables, and fiber.

These foods cannot deliver the nutrition that we require for healthy, properly functioning bodies and immune systems. They are largely stripped of their nutrition during processing, and what nutrition remains is of low quality.

Even though you are eating a sufficient number of calories, your body may actually be in a state of starvation, because it is deprived of these crucial micronutrients. The SAD makes us feel full, but since the calories we are eating are lacking in real nutrition, we may feel driven to eat even more as our bodies seek the nutrition that they so desperately need.

Most often, overweight people are starving at the cellular level!

A quick peek into your pantry and refrigerator will tell you if you are eating this SAD diet. Cereals, white pastas, packaged and processed foods, chips, cookies cakes—all these are evidence of the SAD. If, however, you find mostly vegetables and high-quality proteins, along with some fruits and complex carbohydrates, chances are you are on the right track.

However, no matter how diligent you are to eat the proper balance of foods, it is hard to ensure that you are getting the right amount of micronutrients. Even the nutrients in healthy foods vary depending on the season and the health of the soil in which they were grown.

Study after study has shown that we simply cannot get all the nutrients our bodies need from food alone—even if we eat the best-quality organic food. That's where proper supplementation comes in.

Unfortunately, there are countless supplement companies on the market that are more concerned with making a profit than making an actual difference. Multiple investigations over the years have shown that many of these products don't even contain the ingredients claimed on the label! The reality is that most products that do actually contain said ingredients (in a reasonable amount to have benefit) lack the delivery system to even make the supplements useful to your body.

Choosing the Right Supplements for You

Rather than give you a list of recommended supplements, we want to address choosing the right brand of supplements.

First, understand the old saying, "You get what you pay for." That's not to say you have to buy the most expensive supplements on the market, but you do need to pay attention and steer clear of the cheap stuff. There's a big difference between what you get with a multivitamin that costs only $7 for a month's supply and one that costs $50.

Next, when we purchase food we prefer to go with local as much as possible. You can really tell the difference in the freshness, taste, and quality of the food. Now, with supplements, typically local is not an option. However, knowing the people behind the supplements, or at least knowing someone you trust who knows the people behind the supplements, is ideal. By the way, home shopping networks, celebrity-endorsed products, and your favorite daytime talk show host are probably not the best sources.

Finally, you have to look beyond the colorful brochures and fancy websites. Dig down into how the supplements are manufactured. Choose a company that has a solid foundation rooted in innovation, quality, safety, and effectiveness.

TIPS FOR DINING OUT & TRAVEL

Food is a significant part of why we enjoy traveling. Since we travel often, we don't eat out much when we're home. We do enjoy the food where we are visiting, but we focus on seeking out the highest-quality food possible. We also make conscious decisions about which foods are truly "worth it." Gelato in Italy was absolutely 100 percent worth it! Every bite was eaten slowly and thoroughly enjoyed. For us, alcohol is never worth it and anything that contains gluten is rarely worth it.

It has taken us practice to get to a place where we can pause and make conscious decisions concerning foods that are less healthy, and when we do choose to eat them, to be guilt and regret free. It has taken time to be able to stop and not allow indulgence to send us down a path of less healthy food for days. This will take time and practice, and you won't always get it right.

Dining Out

Dining out can be stressful if you are watching what you eat. Here are some guidelines to make it more enjoyable and still stay on course:

- **Limit the number of times you eat out.** You have much more control over the quality of food and how it is prepared when you are home. You can also make something for a fraction of the cost of going out to eat!

- **Ask questions and plan ahead.** Research where you're eating, and don't be afraid to ask if you can go to a particular restaurant where you will to have good options. When you are placing your order, be sure to ask questions about how your food is prepared, such as the oils used for cooking.

- **Order first!** This will keep you from being tempted to waver from your original order. Studies show that the first person to order can and will set the stage for how the rest of the table orders. Set a good example.

- **Skip the breadbasket, if possible.** It is much easier to not consume any bread if you don't have to stare at it the entire time you wait for your meal.

- **Be cautious of marinades, sauces, and breading.** These likely contain gluten, sugar, soy, or other hidden ingredients.

- **Ask for substitutions.** Most meals will come with some kind of starch or grain. Ask to substitute with steamed vegetables or a salad.

- **Bring your own fats or dressings.** If you're going to eat a salad, try bringing your own dressing. You can make a great dressing with olive oil, lemon juice, and a bit of salt.

- **Any restaurant you go to can accommodate you.** Ask for a plain serving of protein, steamed/cooked vegetables instead of grains or starches, and/or a salad without croutons or dressing. If you don't have dressing with you, ask for olive oil and lemons to make your own. Most salad dressing will contain gluten, soybean oil, and/or canola oil.

- **Ask for a gluten-free menu.** This is a good place to start. From there you can ask for steamed vegetables or a salad for a side. When we eat out we are most concerned with avoiding gluten, as that is what we will have the largest reaction to. For others, it may be important to pay attention to dairy or inflammatory cooking oils.

Travel

Travel often brings eating plans to a screeching halt, but that isn't necessary. Here are some guidelines to help:

- **If you are driving, prepare a few meals in advance that you don't mind eating cold.** Travel with a cooler to store your food. Examples could be canned fish with avocado or chicken with vegetables and a fat such as coconut oil or ghee. Snacks could include jerky (no added sugar), Dang coconut chips (without added sugar), cut-up vegetables, and fruit.

- **Stay in a place that has a kitchen for food preparation.** You can even make a quick trip to the grocery store and get rotisserie chicken, salad greens, vegetables, and some fruit to store in the fridge.

- **Make sure you eat a nutrient-dense meal** before heading to the airport or pack snacks such as the foods listed above to hold you over until you reach your destination. The airport is the hardest place to find healthy options. When we fly, we always pack a meal or snacks.

What About Cheats & Treats?

The language we use around food can be oh so powerful! You may not think that whether you label a food as good or bad has any bearing on you, but if you really pay attention, our guess is that it plays with your emotions.

Why is it that we use the same word for eating a piece of cake and committing infidelity? What if we stopped using the word "cheat" to attach morality to our food choices? "Cheat" is a word with negative connotations. Labeling foods as "cheats" can get into your heads and be detrimental in your progress of establishing good habits and mind-sets around food.

We used to plan cheat meals into our nutrition program, and then count the days until we could have whatever it was that we considered cheating food—not a great approach to establish healthy eating behaviors. What we found was these cheat meals were anticlimactic and often times when the day and/or meal came, we didn't even want the food but ate it anyway because that is what we had planned to do.

What if you could have any food, any time you wanted? At one point that sounded really scary to us, and maybe it sounds scary to you right now. As you practice intention and mindfulness, you will discover that most often you don't even want these "so-called" *cheat* foods.

Would using the word "treat" be better? We used to think so, but . . .

While the word "treat" does bring about more positive feelings than "cheat," it also implies, *"I have been good so I deserve a treat."* There we go back to labeling ourselves good and bad when it comes to food. There is nothing wrong with treating yourself to a massage or a pedicure, but when it comes to food, this could be a potentially problematic mind-set.

Food should not carry a label with it that equates to good or bad. Let's call food what it is: food. Identifying foods as "less healthy" or "less optimal" is a way for us to differentiate between foods that we know do not support or contribute to our health and well-being. For example, a plate of whole wheat pasta is less healthy than using zucchini noodles or spaghetti squash as a substitution.

Not labeling certain foods as treats allows you to provide yourself with self-care "treats" that are not food, like a massage or an afternoon alone enjoying a good book. Those activities will restore and rejuvenate you much more than would a cupcake or pizza and beer.

PART 3

THE TRAINING PROGRAM

chapter 14

STOP EXERCISING IF YOU WANT LONG-TERM RESULTS

So you're ready to start exercising. Well, here's where we tell you *not* to.

Huh?

Here are the hard facts:

- Weight loss is the number-one New Year's resolution in the US each year . . .

- Only 46 percent of people kept their resolutions beyond six months—*most quit within the first month!*

- Only 8 percent achieved their goals!

Success is a mind-set that very few of us possess. That's why we opened this book with an entire chapter dedicated to mind-set. We all have the same twenty-four hours in the day, but only a select few have the mental discipline to truly change their circumstances within those twenty-four hours.

So, if you truly want better health and fitness, we're going to have to shift your mind-set by telling you to "stop exercising!"

Yes, we're serious. We want you to *stop exercising*. To reach and maintain your goals, you must start *training*.

There's a *serious* difference. Exercise may or may not be fun, but you've convinced yourself to do it today because you perceive that the effect you produce is of benefit to you today. This is where group fitness classes, boot camps, and even DVDs you buy from late-night TV come into play. They provide you with exercises to do—you'll "feel the burn," get your heart pumping, and even stimulate muscle growth. You will see some results just because you went from nothing to something.

Training, on the other hand, has a specific plan, purpose, and reason. It's related to what you did yesterday and part of a plan to do tomorrow and *it's individualized to you*. It's big-picture thinking and incorporates specific exercises done in specific ways at specific times within the overall plan.

Now, we don't want to downplay the benefits of these *random* workouts; we'd much rather see you show up to the most poorly put together group exercise class (as long as it's not hurting you) than do nothing at all. However, we're assuming that you want a *program with a purpose*, and you want to make a *transformation* over the next six weeks and beyond.

If that sounds great to you, let's get into your training program...

CASE STUDY: **TRAINING WITH VISION**

I played volleyball, softball, danced, ran, and rode bike (lots of cardio). I even taught step aerobics in college. I was actively moving my body, but my weight never really changed. I was going through the motions of physical activity without purpose or intensity.

Then I had children and wanted to "exercise" off the baby weight. I returned to running and riding a bike. Unfortunately, I became discouraged because my exercise efforts were not bringing the results I was hoping for. I was beginning to feel defeated and almost ready to accept that the body I was in was as good as it was going to get. Being a competitive person, I knew I couldn't settle for "good enough." I needed a different approach.

Transformation Club taught me about real training. I was a bit skeptical because I didn't want to become a bodybuilder. I did want be stronger and healthier. I didn't really think I had anything to train for. As I began training with intensity and focus, my view changed. I had a new desire for measurable change, and training brought those changes faster than I had ever experienced just exercising. I was powered by a healthy vision of myself. Training gave me a purpose, and I lost twenty pounds in six weeks. I had never lost that much weight with the years of cardio I was doing previously. I dropped six dress sizes and felt stronger than I had ever been in my entire life. High-intensity interval training jump-started my metabolism and increased my endurance. It made me stronger and more confident. I have been able to reach my fitness goals in a shorter amount of time due to the focus and potency of training. The results ignited my motivation. Training has also helped the weight stay off. I realized I do have something to train for . . . life!

—Shelly Kasid

TRAINING PROGRAM CONSIDERATIONS

One of the truly unique aspects of our training programs is our program scheduling. We certainly didn't invent this concept, but you typically only find it in sports-conditioning programs.

While most group fitness programs design their workouts week-to-week or even day-to-day, we design our workouts annually! Yes, every workout is pre-programmed to ensure a proper training "flow" that provides our members the best (and most sustainable) results possible.

This process is referred to as **periodization**. Periodization employs phase-specific variations of training, each with a specific goal or training adaptation. Periodization systematically overloads the body to create a desired physical change (strength gains, muscle development, fat loss, endurance, etc.), while balancing work and rest to avoid overtraining, burnout, and/or injury. Ultimately, the annual training program (**macrocycle**) aims at achieving the best possible, long-term results for our clients . . .

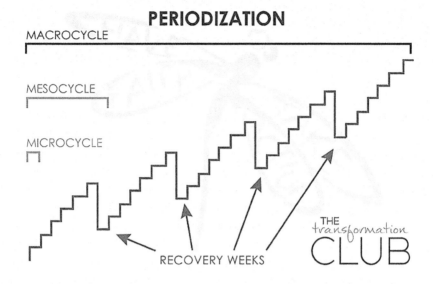

Think of it this way—athletes have different *seasons* in their overall training program and their workouts must be adjusted accordingly. For example, the post-season would likely incorporate a lot of rehab work before moving into the off-season, which would be more about building up strength and perhaps size. Pre-season would focus on gameplay conditioning, and in-season would be about maintenance, getting through the season injury free, and getting to the playoffs in peak condition. Those seasons would be further broken down into different training programs (e.g., a four-month off-season might break down into four four-week programs that progress as you go along).

While we don't have a seasonal flow with an annual end goal (championship) in mind, we do want to structure our program with the intent of improving how we look, feel, and perform throughout the year, and then year-to-year. Like a fine wine, we want to improve with age!

CASE STUDY: **TRAINING FOR TRANSFORMATION**

I have worked out at several gyms—big and small. The Transformation Club was the first one that my fitness level was assessed before beginning to workout. I knew I had found a safe place! I was diagnosed with rheumatoid arthritis years ago and didn't think I could workout on a regular basis. One day things were fine, the next day I couldn't move.

I was accepted at The Transformation Club as a challenger in July and so began my journey back to fitness. My assessment indicated I had shoulder and knee issues, so every workout I do alternative exercises. I felt a sense of accomplishment following each workout. Although it is group training, the coaches work with each person and help everyone work to their personal best. It is so rewarding to get through a workout and know I have done my best. I have gotten so strong in five months and feel more empowered than ever in my life. The Club trainers and staff are supportive and relentless about form and safety in training. The fear of tomorrow is gone for me, and I will continue to train with the Transformation Club under their most outstanding guidance.

—LuAnn Nead

Mesocycles

We have found that dividing our annual training program into eight **mesocycles** works well for our members. Each mesocycle is six weeks in length, although at our training facility there is some variation (based on the holiday/school calendar), for convenience.

Each cycle is programmed with a specific training adaption—strength, muscle gain, endurance, or fat loss—in mind, taking into account the different muscle fiber types and energy systems we have in our bodies.

Now, let's be clear; there will be side benefits to each cycle—working in a strength development phase will also increase fat loss, decrease joint pain, and boost energy—it's just that our primary focus for that phase is strength. By the way, if your primary goal is weight/fat loss, then you can't just follow a fat/weight-loss training protocol. You *will* hit a plateau. That's where following a well-put-together training program comes in.

Microcycles

A **microcycle** is a week of training. Each week might consist of two, three, four, or more different training sessions, and are often labeled Workout A, Workout B, Workout C, etc.

A three-day training protocol on Mondays, Wednesdays, and Fridays, for example would simply be A/B/C. For years, we've had great success with this schedule. We also have what could be called a Workout D on Saturdays but not in the traditional sense because it varies week to week.

These training sessions are performed for the duration of the mesocycle. This is an important training philosophy–don't be fooled by clever marketing gimmicks. We don't want to confuse your muscles, we want to develop them, make them stronger, and more metabolic, ultimately burning loads of unwanted fat and shaping a strong, slim, and sexy body! This can only be accomplished through repetition. As you become more skilled at the workouts each week, you'll be able to recruit more muscle fibers, do more weight and repetitions, and see greater results.

TRAINING SESSIONS

Each training session has a specific purpose in the program, as well. During some mesocycles (for a metabolic resistance training program, for example), each training session in the microcycle (A/B/C for example) will incorporate the same exercise-to-work ratio. This is a more traditional approach to interval training. A classic example would be Tabata training. Each of the workouts would incorporate 20:10 (twenty seconds of work, ten seconds of rest) intervals for eight rounds.

Other times, the training sessions will incorporate different exercise-to-work ratios. This is known as undulating interval training. That might look something like this:

- Workout A: 15:45 power intervals

- Workout B: 30:30 strength intervals

- Workout C: 45:15 endurance intervals

Both methods are beneficial and have their place in an overall training program.

RECOVERY WEEK

One of the most important (but misunderstood) secrets to smart training programs is the necessity of taking a break. Taking a break means *stopping all exercise for several days or even a whole week.* Exercising every day with no breaks can be detrimental to your overall fitness progress and cause *overtraining*. When you overtrain, you do not give your body time to recover and heal from the stress you place on it while exercising.

- **Overtraining makes you more vulnerable to muscle strain and injury.** During intense exercise, small tears in your muscles occur (that's normal). You may also from time to time notice a sore joint or some stiffness. Typically, these small inconveniences settle down with a good night's rest and an ice pack. But over time, these slight "injuries" can accumulate and intensify because your body doesn't get enough time off to fully recover. The result can be a full-blown injury that takes you out of training altogether!

- **Your nervous system needs a break, too.** Following an intense workout schedule week after week takes its toll on your nervous system. When your nervous system gets overloaded, you may find that you feel irritable, weak, and unmotivated. If you continue to ignore your body's plea for recovery, you will probably find that your symptoms only worsen. Then your workouts will suffer (yielding poor or no results), you'll likely end up sick, or worse—end up quitting due to burnout.

- Whether you are working for fat loss, muscle strength, cardio improvement, or a combination of all three, recovery is vital. *Your body must have a break from the stress.*

COMMON SYMPTOMS OF NEEDING TIME OFF INCLUDE:

- an actual injury or illness

- persistent soreness

- a halt in progression—hitting a plateau that won't budge

- feeling bored, unmotivated, and/or dreading your workouts

- general fatigue

- a higher than normal morning pulse

- insomnia

- lack of appetite

DELOADING

Deloading is essentially a recovery training protocol where you significantly reduce the amount of work performed in each session. You might simply cut all your weights in half and go through the motions, focusing on improving/mastering your technique. This will reduce the stress on your body but still keep you moving throughout the week, keeping your body active and helping it recover with increased blood flow. Another approach to deloading (one we generally recommend) is to change up the workouts for the week with long walks, yoga, specific recovery workouts, etc.

STOP EXERCISING IF YOU WANT LONG-TERM RESULTS

You need to listen to your body. Many times, it's more beneficial to sleep in (if you normally workout early in the morning) or kick back and read a good book during your normal training time to give your body the recovery it needs.

Remember, there is a tremendous amount of thought and preparation that goes into designing a solid training program with a long-term approach to success. But doing something is usually better than doing nothing—doing random exercise consistently is far better than sitting on your hands because you're too confused to start or you're waiting for the perfect program.

MINIMUM EFFECTIVE LOADING

There is a common misunderstanding regarding exercise—*"more is better."* It's kind of like the old saying, *"No pain. No gain."*

Both are completely *false* when it comes to exercise for weight loss, fitness, and even performance.

There is a right and wrong way to approach your exercise program. That's where MEL comes in.

Minimum Effective Load (MEL) is a term created by Arthur Jones, inventor of Nautilus® exercise machines. Jones defined the minimum effective load as "the smallest load needed to get the desired outcome."[31] Doing any more is simply wasted effort at best and detrimental to results or even harmful at worst.

This same approach can be applied to how often you exercise and how hard you push yourself. And it's not just limited to weight lifting exercises. It applies to all forms of exercise, although then it's generally referred to as Minimum Effective Dosage (MED).

---

31   "Weight Loss: Metabolism and Weight Loss: How You Burn Calories," n.p., October 6, 2011. accessed May 6, 2014.

It is important to realize that no matter who you are, overtraining will not deliver faster and better results. Instead, it will lead to injury and/or burnout. Your wisest choice is to practice moderation and consistency using the MEL and MED principles.

"HOW MUCH EXERCISE IS ENOUGH?"

We have all heard the obesity statistics and they're atrocious, so let's simply get down to what works to lose weight and get fit. Going from nothing to something is, well, something. If you haven't been exercising for twenty years and you decide to dust off the old workout shoes, just going through the motions and *performing corrective exercises* three times per week is a *great* start!

You simply don't need to do *insane* workout DVDs to get a good workout. In fact, it will ultimately be detrimental in the long run.

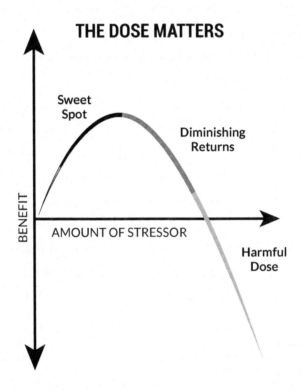

THE DOSE MATTERS

Sweet Spot

Diminishing Returns

BENEFIT

AMOUNT OF STRESSOR

Harmful Dose

While many folks will initially lose weight if they engage in sixty minutes of nonstop daily exercise, any gains will eventually be eroded by factors like burnout, injury, and boredom. Exceeding the minimum effective dosage does *not* deliver greater results—quite the opposite, in fact.

This reality is exemplified by conclusions drawn from a 2009 study performed on sedentary, overweight, postmenopausal women that forced a dramatic increase in the amount and intensity of their daily exercise: "…we observed no difference in the actual and predicted weight loss with 4 and 8 KKW of exercise (72 and 136 minutes respectively), while the 12 KKW (194 minutes) produced only about half of the predicted weight loss."[32]

Author Tim Ferriss writes in *The 4-Hour Body*, *"More is not better. Indeed, your greatest challenge will be resisting the temptation to do more."*[33] If on your exercise journey you blast out of the gate at top speed with an intensity that you can't possibly sustain, you will burn out and likely give up.

Remember, what you do every day is more important than what you do every once in a while. Those everyday activities may not be terribly exciting while you are doing them; they may not feel like you are making progress but give the compound effect time to work. Your effort will pay off. You will become leaner, stronger, more fit, and others will begin to notice.

Take care of your body and your mind by practicing the minimum effective dosage strategy and you will achieve your goals… for life!

32   T.S., Martin, C.K., Thompson, A.M., Earnest, C. P. Catherine, R. M., Blair, S. N. "Changes in weight, waist circumference and compensatory responses with different doses of exercise among sedentary, overweight postmenopausal women." PLoS ONE 4(2): e4515. Doi: 10.1371/journal.pone.004515.)
33   Timothy Ferris, *The 4-Hour Body* (New York: Crown Publishers, 2010), 18–19.

chapter 15

RESISTANCE TRAINING

We could write an entire book on this one subject and put it right next to all the others on the shelves at Barnes & Noble that argue their referenced approach to resistance training as the end-all, be-all method. The truth is, they're all effective and incorporating each of them at different points in your training can be ideal.

At the most basic level, you can think of resistance training like this: you're working your muscles against resistance (your own body weight or an external load provided by a resistance band, dumbbell, or kettlebell) in an effort to increase power and strength, build muscle, increase endurance, and improve performance.

To make things more confusing, each of those goals (power, strength, muscle, etc.) can be accomplished with a variety of different approaches to strength training. Again, you'll find shelves full of books, each arguing their method as the best. We won't worry about that right now.

Instead, let's focus on the long list of benefits resistance training provides.

RESISTANCE TRAINING AND MUSCLE MASS

As we age, muscle mass loss is inevitable without regular strength training workouts. Muscle tissue is not easy tissue to gain back. This is especially true for women who naturally have low amounts of testosterone compared to men. Protecting muscle you already have is one of the most important considerations of any well-rounded fitness program.

If you begin losing muscle mass, your strength will decrease, meaning everyday activities—including those outdoor activities you want to take part in—will become harder and harder.

Muscle also plays a major role in fat burning. While exercise does burn calories, you only work out a few hours per week. To increase fat burning you need to increase your metabolism, specifically your Resting Metabolic Rate (RMR). Those who have a higher degree of muscle mass burn more calories even when they're at rest.[34] As a person ages, metabolism naturally slows down, leading to gradual weight gain. Muscle is a great way to counterbalance the body's natural slowdown, and the earlier a person starts, the easier it will be to maintain that muscle over time.

34   "U.S. National Library of Medicine, "Aging Changes in the Bones–Muscles– Joints," *MedlinePlus*, 2012, https://medlineplus.gov/ency/article/004015.htm.

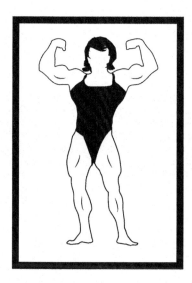

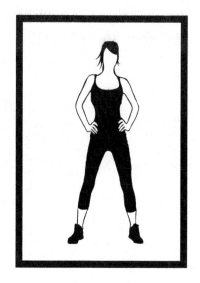

What women think
they'll look like if they
lift heavy weights

What will
actually happen

Many people complain that the reason they're gaining weight into their forties and fifties is due to a slow metabolism, but really, that slow metabolism is happening (partly) because they are losing muscle. The muscle gains you achieve with a proper strength-training program can help reverse this process and actually *increase* metabolism!

Will resistance training make me big and bulky?

No! The fact is, it's not easy to add large amounts of muscle to our bodies. Adding large amounts of muscle requires very specific training and nutrition protocols, and, in most cases, performance-enhancing drugs—this is especially true for women.

Look at it this way: one pound of muscle is about the size of your hand when you make a fist. Distributed across your body, it is nearly unnoticeable.

Adding five to ten pounds of muscle will dramatically improve your shape (in a great way), health, and performance. Life is much better with a little more muscle.

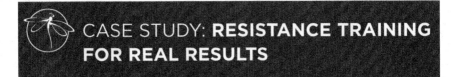

CASE STUDY: **RESISTANCE TRAINING FOR REAL RESULTS**

Cardio equals weight loss, right? That's what I always thought. When I felt it was time to lose some weight I would join a gym, spend forty-five minutes on the treadmill several times a week, cut down on how much I was eating, and voila! I expected the weight to fall off.

That was never the case. I was sweaty, exhausted, and "hangry" (hungry *and* angry), and the scale would barely move. To spend all that time starving and running (which I hate with a passion) was frustrating. Eventually I would stop going to the gym and resumed my normal eating habits. And running wasn't the only thing I tried. I was always searching for the miracle cardio cure, from Zumba to Hip Hop Abs. I wanted to find a way to lose weight that was both fun and sustainable, but each new venture would last a couple weeks, and then I would lose interest.

I was pretty sedentary during my second pregnancy and gained quite a bit of weight. When my son was born, I was ready for change. I didn't look like *me* anymore. This wasn't *my* body! That's when Justin and Janell introduced me to resistance training. I'll have to admit, in my first couple weeks with them I was skeptical about how this type of training would lead to weight loss. I still thought I needed to sweat profusely to lose weight. Boy was I wrong. Between changing what I was eating and adding the resistance training, the weight started to fall off. In less than six months, I lost fifty-five pounds. It was awesome!

And one of the most important things is that I *love* this way of training because it's efficient and fun. I actually get excited for training days! Who doesn't want a super effective training session in thirty minutes? I hated spending over an hour at the gym. And there's so much you can do with resistance training, I could never imagine getting bored.

I am now at the same weight I was on my wedding day, except I wear two sizes smaller! Why? Because when I was losing weight before, it was in a very unhealthy way. I still had a lot of body fat instead of muscle, so my body was more "fluffy." With resistance training, I have built up lean muscle, which is more compact and makes my body firm. I'm stronger and leaner than I have ever been in my life. Some days I still can't believe this is *my* body, but now it's in a good way!

—Lindsay Belden

RESISTANCE TRAINING AND BONE HEALTH

As a person grows older, bone loss is inevitable, especially for women after menopause.[35] This can cause bones to break more easily, feelings of fatigue and weakness, and reduced tolerance to physical activity.

Weight-bearing exercises strengthen bones, help minimize natural bone loss, and reduce the risk of injury.[36]

While other outdoor activities may be weight bearing in nature and still help with bone strength and formation, no other exercise is more weight bearing than is strength training.

Since you'll be supporting more weight than just your body weight, you can really take your bone health to the next level. One study published in the journal of *Medicine and Science in Sports and Exercise* illustrated that strength training is superior in terms of combating osteoporosis, compared to aerobic activity only.[37]

This can prevent stress fractures or bone breaks down the road, both of which could become very serious if you are into your sixties and seventies.

RESISTANCE TRAINING AND DISEASE PREVENTION

Strength training has been shown to provide a number of health benefits, including a reduced risk of cardiovascular disease and diabetes.[38]

---

35   U.S. National Library of Medicine, "Build Up Your Bones," *MedlinePlus*, 2011, https://medlineplus.gov/magazine/issues/winter11/articles/winter11pg15.html
36   "Why Strength Training?" Centers for Disease Control and Prevention (Feb. 24, 2011).
37   J. L. Ivy, W. M. Sherman, and W. J. Miller, "Effect of Strength Training on Glucose Tolerance and Post-Glucose Insulin Response," Medicine and Science in Sports and Exercise 16(6): 539–543.
38   "Why Strength Training?" Centers for Disease Control and Prevention.

A Tufts University study even found that participants in a strength-training program were able to see a marked reduction in arthritis pain. In fact, the study found that the end result was better than that received from medications.

Strength training can also improve a person's mental health, reducing depression and improving sleep quality.

RESISTANCE TRAINING AND INSULIN SENSITIVITY

Lastly, strength training can positively impact insulin sensitivity. Your insulin sensitivity level is one of the key factors determining your risk of diabetes and metabolic syndrome, a condition that's starting to impact more and more females.

A regular strength-training workout routine will help to keep your tissue cells more responsive to insulin. Should you consume carbohydrates in your diet, your body will be able to better utilize those carbohydrates, directing them toward the muscle cells rather than the body fat cells.[39]

This also helps keep you leaner, since you'll have a reduced rate of converting those carbohydrates into body fat stores. It appears the primary reason for this is due to the increased lean muscle tissue development, which then increases the insulin sensitivity level.

Each of these benefits helps you to live healthier, enjoying a better quality of life and longevity. However, we understand that a big reason you're reading this book is because you want to make a physical transformation. Don't worry, strength training is going to play a major role in that, too! Think of strength training as your tool for building and sculpting your strong, slim, and sexy body.

---

39 Ivy, J.L., Sherman, W.M., and Miller, W.J., "Effect of strength training on glucose tolerance and post-glucose insulin response." *Medicine and Science in Sports and Exercise* 16, no. 6 (1984), 539–543.

RESISTANCE TRAINING METHODS

Traditionally, the cornerstone of most resistance training programs has been performing exercises in a **straight set format**—a specified number or reps for a given exercise, rest for thirty seconds to a few minutes, and then repeat before moving on to the next exercise. Fat-loss and endurance programs typically prescribe shorter rest periods, whereas strength and power programs prescribe longer rest periods.

So what's the problem with this format? There really isn't one if you look at it from a stimulus-response standpoint. In other words, it *does* produce results!

However, this approach to resistance training can get boring quickly; for most people, that means the end of the program. It can also be time consuming. You pump out your ten reps, go to the water fountain, chat with some friends, check Facebook, and then go back to the bar to pump out set number two. By the time you're done with your fourth set, it's taken you almost ten minutes to complete only one exercise. It's no wonder people are spending ninety minutes to two hours in the gym!

Ninety percent of members who join a health club do so to lose weight and look better. If you're reading this book, you probably fall into that category (although by now you understand that a *transformation* is so much more than that). You're probably short on time, too.

ALTERNATING SETS

A more effective, time-efficient approach is the **alternating set format**. Here you'll perform one exercise, rest for a short period of time, then perform another noncompeting exercise, rest for a short period of time, and so forth.

Alternating sets allows you to work different areas of your body when you would otherwise be resting with the straight set format. Plus, by working another area of your body with a noncompeting exercise, you allow your body to recover from the previous exercise(s). The result is improved training economy and density: more work accomplished in less time, the cornerstone of any sound fat-loss program. There are a number of different ways to perform alternating sets:

- Supersets: Alternate between two different noncompeting exercises (e.g., upper body and lower body, such as push-ups and lunges, or upper body push and upper body pull, such as chest press and rows).

- Trisets: Alternate between three different exercises (e.g., push, pull, and lower body such as push-ups, rows, and lunges, or upper body, lower body, "core" such as chin-up, deadlift, plank).

- Circuits: Alternate between four or more different exercises.

AN EXAMPLE WORKOUT CONSISTING OF ALTERNATING SETS IS:

- 1A) Resistance band Romanian deadlifts
- 1B) Push-ups
  - Perform eight to ten reps of each exercise four times through.
- 2A) KB goblet squats
- 2B) Suspension trainer rows

- Perform six to eight reps of each exercise four times through.
  - ▫ 3A) Dumbbell curl plus overhead press
  - ▫ 3B) Ab wheel rollouts
    - Perform ten to twelve reps of each exercise three times through.

HIGH-INTENSITY TRAINING

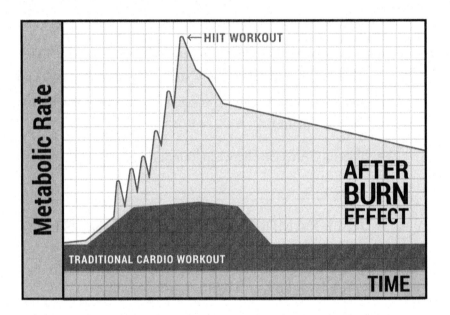

High-intensity interval training (HIIT) is an exercise strategy that employs an intense bout of exercise followed by a brief rest. HIIT protocols use a variety of work to rest ratios that generally consist of five to ten cycles per circuit and workouts consist of four to six circuits lasting twenty to thirty minutes, although there are even benefits to performing just one circuit for a quick five-minute workout.

HIIT workouts were originally performed as a cardiovascular training method (sprint workouts, for example) but have become more popular as a method of resistance training—generally referred to as **metabolic resistance training (MRT).**

HIIT workouts, especially MRT workouts are incredibly effective for our busy members seeking a body transformation with just a few short workouts per week. The results we've seen have been amazing!

HIIT accomplishes this in the following ways:

- **Creates the optimal hormonal environment for fat loss:** HIIT puts your body in a "fight or flight" mode.[40] As a result, your body releases certain hormones that directly mobilize stored fat to be burned off as energy during exercise.

- **Burn a *ton* of calories both during and after exercise:** Excess post-exercise oxygen consumption (EPOC), otherwise known as post-workout "after-burn," is a measurably increased rate of oxygen intake after strenuous activity. This after-burn creates an elevated metabolic rate for twenty-four to forty-eight hours after exercise where fat

---

40   *Fight or flight mode* happens when your body's sympathetic nervous system is stimulated by stress. As noted elsewhere in this book, when your body is under stress, the hormone cortisol is released. Cortisol gets a bad reputation because it is our stress hormone. It's also been dubbed as the "belly fat storing hormone" because excessive cortisol production can lead to increases in belly fat. However, the production of cortisol in short bursts is not the problem. In fact, it's necessary for survival and dealing with acute stressful situations. Cortisol becomes an issue when you're under chronic stress and you stay in fight or flight mode for long periods of time or even all day—as is the case for so many people in today's high-paced, high-stress society.
Part of the benefits of HIIT workouts is that they elicit a positive hormonal response and take advantage of the stress response.

is the primary fuel source. In other words, you burn more fat while you're resting!

- **Increased glycogen storage:** HIIT training rapidly reduces glycogen (stored sugar in the muscle cells) during training. With proper post-workout refueling, your muscle cells "learn" to store more sugar, thus preventing that unwanted sugar-to-fat conversion. Carbs aren't the enemy when they have a place to go other than your butt and gut.

"It Really, Really Works!"

Steven Boutcher, a scientist at the University of South Wales, did a study on high-intensity interval training and found that more fat is lost during shorter, maximum intensity intervals than during slower and longer workout periods.

Obese women were divided into two groups with identical diets but different exercise protocols for fifteen weeks.

The first group exercised three times each week for twenty minutes. Their high-intensity workouts consisted of intervals with eight seconds of max effort and twelve seconds of recovery.

The second group also exercised three times each week, but for forty minutes, and the intensity was steadier.

The results: In spite of the second group's longer exercise periods, the first group saw a higher loss of body fat, especially in the belly, thighs, and hips.

We now know that you can get even better body-shaping results when you perform HIIT using multi-joint strength training exercises like squats, deadlifts, rows, presses, etc. (a.k.a. metabolic resistance training).

What's an example of a HIIT circuit? Here's one of our favorites. It's a six-exercise circuit:

1. Alternating kettlebell snatch

2. Push-ups

3. KB goblet squats

4. Suspension trainer rows

5. Resistance band Romanian deadlifts

6. Burpees

You will alternate between thirty seconds of work and fifteen seconds of rest for all six exercises, followed by one minute of rest. Perform this circuit two to six times, depending on your fitness level and the time you have available.

FINAL THOUGHTS ON RESISTANCE TRAINING METHODS

At the end of the day, all three methods and the countless versions of each will produce results. What matters most is:

- Finding the method(s) that you enjoy and will stick to.

- Varying the methods to avoid plateaus and reap the benefits each provides.

Regular resistance training has many benefits and it's crucial to your transformation, but as with many things, if you take it too far (especially MRT), it can start to have negative consequences. More is not always better.

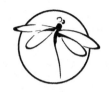

chapter 16

CARDIO TRAINING

Like resistance training, there are many forms of cardio training, each with different outcomes. For the sake of space and relevancy, we're going to address cardio in regard to a physique transformation program—getting strong, slim, and sexy.

Cardiovascular exercise is any exercise that raises your heart rate.

Now, traditionally, when we think of cardio exercises we think of riding a bike, going for a run, or doing whatever it is you do on an elliptical machine. General recommendations are low to moderate intensity (in the "fat burning zone") for sustained periods of time (typically twenty to sixty minutes). Boring!

Of course, you can spice things up a little by doing an aerobics class, but does that make it any more effective?

There's the key thing we need to look at—**effectiveness.**

To determine if your program is effective, you must first go back to your goals.

We're going to focus our cardio training on the following goals:

- Lose weight and/or fat.

- "Tone up."

- Obtain a flatter stomach.

- Get tighter, more defined arms and legs.

- Sculpt a firmer butt.

- Have more energy for work and play.

- Decrease/eliminate joint pain.

- Improve heart and brain health.

Will doing traditional low-to-moderate intensity, long-duration cardio get you those results? How about the "new-school" high-intensity interval training (HIIT) methods? The answer is—maybe.

Maybe?! What kind of answer is that?

First things first—especially for someone just getting started—just about any form/style of exercise is going to be beneficial. If you've been sedentary for the past twenty years, getting out and riding a horse for twenty minutes a day would get you in better shape—and the horse is doing most of the work!

Seriously though, in the beginning it almost doesn't matter what you do, provided it's safe and takes your individual functional capabilities into play. That's why programs like the *Couch to 5K* work so well (at first). Although, I'd argue that most people who do that program or similar programs are setting themselves up for serious injury down the line.

SOME TRUTHS AND MYTHS ABOUT CARDIO

There are a couple different "camps" when it comes to cardio training. There are the endurance nuts who just want to keep piling on the time as if we had nothing else going on in our life. On the other end of the spectrum, there are the four-minute freaks who say you just need to do an HIIT circuit as hard as humanly possible. Let's take a look at the pluses and minuses of each.

The Endurance Training Method

There's no question there are some really lean and fit endurance athletes. However, swing by any local 5k, 10k, or even half marathon and watch the people crossing the finish line. We promise you, a large percentage of those people are overweight, not tone, not firm, not flat, not achieving/sustaining the goals mentioned.

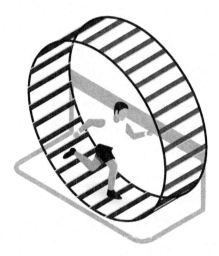

In fact, according to the *Journal of Obesity,* "Most aerobic exercise interventions have consisted of moderate-intensity steady-state exercise, for about thirty to forty min for three to four days per week, over a four- to six-month period. Disappointingly, these kinds of exercise programs have resulted in minimal fat loss." Another study in *Obesity* reports that after logging three hundred hours of cardiovascular exercise (one hour each day, six days per week) over the course of one year, women only lost four pounds and men lost six.[41] That means that for every fifty hours of cardio, you lose only one pound of weight.

Why? Because excessive long-duration cardio can actually *increase* fat storage and decrease lean muscle. One of the biggest reasons is because excessive long-duration cardio places a tremendous amount of stress on your body. When this happens, you end up with a hormonal nightmare—and hormones are what ultimately control everything.

When you're under stress, your cortisol levels get imbalanced, and your thyroid shuts down. Among other things, your thyroid produces T3, which is an important fat-burning hormone. When your T3 is suppressed, your body starts gaining and storing fat immediately.

If all that wasn't enough, cardio increases your appetite. On one side, you have the physiological hunger—your body actually wants more calories, typically in the form of carbohydrates. On the other side, you have the *psychological* hunger—you feel you deserve to eat those crunchy carbs. Many people end up consuming an average of a hundred calories more than they burned during an exercise where they were trying to burn calories!

There's also some evidence that excessive cardio causes oxidative damage and increases free radicals in your body—both nasty things that are bad for your health.

Now, we're not here to disparage all forms of long-duration cardio, as boring as we find it. *Lower-intensity* cardio and some moderate-intensity, long-duration cardio can be extremely beneficial for your health. In addition, this lower-intensity stuff helps you build a solid "aerobic base"—a very important thing for fat loss and fitness. It also

---

41   Anne McTiernan et al., "Exercise Effect on Weight and Body Fat in Men and Women," *Obesity: A Research Journal* 15(6): 1496–1512.

stimulates the parasympathetic branch ("rest and digest" component) of the autonomic nervous system, builds the cardiovascular system, helps relieve anxiety and stress, improves sleep quality, etc.

The High-Intensity Interval Training (HIIT) Method

Ever since the (often misunderstood) Tabata study was done, people have been jumping on the four-minute workout bandwagon. There's even a certification for it now!

By the way, here's the quick definition of a *true* Tabata workout:

- One exercise performed at *maximum* intensity for twenty seconds followed by ten seconds of rest.

- Repeat for eight brutal rounds.

When you're done, you should be breathless and your lungs should feel like they're on fire. Basically, you should be miserable *but in a good way!*

To learn more about Tabatas, visit www.TheTransformationClub.fitness/Tabatas.

The reality is that most people can't perform a *true* Tabata workout. They simply can't generate enough intensity. That's why a more conventional approach is to use alternating exercises, still at a high (but tolerable) intensity, and perform four to six circuits.

So, the good news about high-intensity interval training (HIIT) is that it is very effective at helping you achieve your goals, especially when done with resistance training exercises.

Is there a downside to HIIT?

Absolutely. Consistent, high-intensity training of any kind will eventually lead to burnout and/or injury. That's one reason why we program recovery weeks into our training program.

NOW WHAT?

Let's start putting all of this into a training program.

Reviewing our goals:

- Lose weight and/or fat.

- "Tone up."

- Obtain a flatter stomach.

- Get tighter, more defined arms and legs.

- Sculpt a firmer butt.

- Have more energy for work and play.

- Decrease/eliminate joint pain.

- Improve heart and brain health.

We're going to get the most bang for our buck from resistance training, specifically metabolic resistance training. What really makes this kind of training perfect for fat burning are the short rests and alternating, noncompeting exercises. MRT done right will get your heart pumping while stimulating sexy lean muscle development! You can truly get the best of both worlds.

Step 1

Incorporate three to four days per week of MRT (and/or other resistance training methods).

If you're not feeling like you're getting enough cardio from your MRT sessions, it's simply because you aren't working hard enough! Unless you're doing a corrective exercise, you need to *get after it!*

Step 2

Now that you're committed to working hard three to four days per week on a consistent basis, you may be saying, *"I feel like I need to do more."*

If you *want* to do more, great. If you *feel* like you need to do more, we must first look at the rest of the picture.

More exercise (resistance or cardio) is not always the answer.

Before we recommend anyone add more to their training program, we first want to know what's going on with their nutrition program, not to mention their sleep patterns and stress management.

If you have a couple extra hours to devote per week to doing cardio on top of your resistance training, and you're not eating real, unprocessed, whole-foods with plenty of lean muscle-building protein, healthy fats, and nutritious vegetables, then we're going to tell you straight-up—**forget about more workouts and get your butt in the kitchen!**

Let's say you're currently training M/W/F mornings. Instead of adding T/Th to the mix to do some cardio, get up and prep a few days' worth of food in that time. You'll get *much better* results from the time you spend in the kitchen than from the time you spend on a treadmill!

Step 3

So far you have three to four awesome resistance-training sessions in per week, and your nutrition is dialed in 80–90 percent—we're not asking for 100 percent here. *You can do this!*

If you want to add in some additional exercise, ask yourself: *Am I getting seven to nine hours a night?* If not, we're going to tell you that's where you should be focusing your time.

Step 4

At this point, you might add in some cardio or yoga. It really comes down to your preferences. If you're under a lot of stress, adding in long bouts of cardio or even short HIIT-style workouts will probably just add to the issue. You would be better off with yoga or taking walks. If, on the other hand, things are going well, consider adding some cardio in.

Here's a pretty good rule of thumb for choosing which kind:

If your morning resting heart rate is **above 70 bpm**, choose a lower intensity form of cardio to improve your aerobic base.

If your morning resting heart rate is **below 70 bpm**, *bring on the HIIT*. However, that doesn't mean you have to *kill it!* There are essentially two types of HIIT that focus on different energy systems in your body.

Alactic-aerobic intervals, which are categorized by:

- work periods of six to ten seconds

- rest periods that are five to six times as long as the work period

- performed at a very high intensity or work rate

An example workout would be a ten-second sprint followed by fifty seconds of walking, repeating for fifteen rounds.

Glycolytic intervals, which are categorized by:

- work periods of twenty to ninety seconds

- rest periods that are generally one to three times as long as the work period

- performed at a very high intensity or work rate[42]

An example workout would be thirty seconds of burpees followed by a thirty-second rest and transition to a set of mountain climbers for another thirty seconds, repeating for twenty total rounds (ten of each exercise).

Both are performed at a very high intensity or work rate. However, the alactic-aerobic intervals are shorter bursts with longer recovery periods. This is a great way to "get after it" without building up a ton of lactic acid, beating up your body, and putting high levels of stress on your central nervous system. Alactic-aerobic intervals are a great way to get started with HIIT cardio. They're also a nice way to change things up if most of your HIIT cardio has been the more traditional glycolytic intervals, which is also very effective for our stated goals.

For those wanting to lose fat weight, we've seen tremendous benefit from following up your HIIT session with twenty to thirty minutes of low to moderate intensity steady-state cardio. Some call it "stubborn fat" cardio because it takes advantage of the hormonal shift that occurs after HIIT and has been shown to aid in burning fat, especially in the "stubborn" areas like your hips, belly, and thighs.

Summary

We constantly hear people saying they need to do more cardio. More often than not, cardio is not the answer. Before you consider adding more cardio to your training program, put your *focus and effort* into a solid resistance training program, good nutrition, proper rest, and stress management. Once you've got that dialed in, look at the

---

42   Mike Robertson, "4 Tips for Unconventional Fat Loss," Robertson Training Systems, May 5, 2015, http://robertsontrainingsystems.com/blog/4-tips-for-unconventional-fat-loss/#.

different types of cardio training and decide which one is best for you at your current fitness level.

We design our workouts with the six-day-per-week member in mind. (Sundays are for long walks with your dog or playing with your kids.) Many people we work with prefer the benefits that come with a daily exercise habit so we carefully design our workouts to give them a great blend of resistance and cardio training without the worry of overtraining. Plus, we have yoga available for those who would see a better result or just prefer performing something more restorative in between their resistance training days.

OTHER TRAINING METHODS TO CONSIDER

The focus of the training portion of this book is on resistance training and cardio training; however, there are other things to consider in an overall training program. For example, you might find yoga to be a very beneficial (and enjoyable) addition to your training program—Janell certainly does, as do many of our members at The Transformation Club.

Yoga is a Hindu spiritual and ascetic discipline, a part of which, including breath control, simple meditation, and the adoption of specific bodily postures, is widely practiced for health and relaxation.

The benefits of yoga are vast. They include but are not limited to:

- helping you move better and feel less stiff or tired

- helping you to build strength and endurance, especially core strength

- helping your body awareness and, therefore, possibly also improving your posture

- feeling less stressed and more relaxed

- helping to lower blood pressure and slow your heart rate

- helping to lower cholesterol and lower triglyceride levels and better immune system function

It doesn't matter if you're twenty-five or sixty-five, able to touch your toes or not, a busy professional or stay-at-home mom. If you can breathe, yoga is for you.

Studies have shown that just one yoga class can significantly reduce tension, anxiety, depression, and fatigue. Sixty minutes of yoga can be as restful and restorative to your body as four hours of sleep!

Yoga calms your mind and lets you glide through life with more control. Plus, yoga can melt away belly fat. That's because stress is a huge factor in fat accumulating around your stomach. As your stress disappears, so does fat!

> *Redeem a free yoga session at*
> *The Transformation Club by visiting*
> *www.TheClubYogaVIP.com.*

The contents of this book are not meant to be a complete guide to creating a total transformation to become the best version of you. There are simply too many variables for each of us to say, "This is the only way to do it."

You may also consider adding in additional stability, mobility, and/ or flexibility training to your weekly routine. You may find that adding in some group fitness classes like kickboxing or spinning are beneficial, or you might have a favorite dance DVD that you like to do.

We're certainly in favor of you participating in activities that you enjoy that could enhance your transformation results. However, we believe (and have seen) that when it comes to the training portion of your transformation plan, resistance training, as outlined in this book, should be the foundation.

It's okay, and even encouraged, to continue with (or add in) your favorite activities, so long as they fit in with your transformation goals and compliment the program we're outlining for you. Just be sure not to overtrain.

chapter 17

SETTING UP YOUR TRAINING SCHEDULE

Helping you create a *customized* training schedule through a book is nearly impossible—there are just so many variables, at the most basic level.

Since we can't know that information for everyone reading this book, we're going to outline a few options, one of which is likely to fit well into your schedule; if not, we'll give you some ideas on how to modify.

In a perfect world, you would be active daily. That does not mean you need to lift weights daily or train with maximum intensity in every session. In fact, that's generally a recipe for overtraining.

THREE-DAY SCHEDULE

Most people can commit to following a three-day-per-week training schedule. In this case, you might follow a three-day rotation (A/B/C) that lays out like this:

SUN	MON	TUE	WED	THU	FRI	SAT
Active Rest	Resistance Training: Total Body	Active Rest	Resistance Training: Total Body	Active Rest	Resistance Training: Total Body	Active Rest

However, don't feel constrained by the days of the week. You can adjust the program to fit just about anything. For example:

SUN	MON	TUE	WED	THU	FRI	SAT
Active Rest	Resistance Training: Upper Body	Resistance Training: Lower Body	Active Rest	Resistance Training: Total Body	Active Rest	Active Rest

Or:

SUN	MON	TUE	WED	THU	FRI	SAT
Active Rest	Resistance Training: Push Muscles	Resistance Training: Pull Muscles	Active Rest	Resistance Training: Total Body	Active Rest	Active Rest

As you can see, with slight modifications (switching from total body to a split routine) we can make just about anything work.

FOUR-DAY SCHEDULE

Let's take a look at a four-day-week training schedule:

SUN	MON	TUE	WED	THU	FRI	SAT
Active Rest	Resistance Training: Upper Body	Resistance Training: Lower Body	Active Rest	Resistance Training: Upper Body	Resistance Training: Lower Body	Active Rest

In this case, we're following an A/B format where Workout A focuses on upper body and Workout B focuses on lower body. You could also do push muscles for A and pull muscles for B—a common favorite for A/B splits.

ADD TO SCHEDULE

Let's say you want to follow one of the thee-day formats and add in your favorite cycling class. That could look like this:

SUN	MON	TUE	WED	THU	FRI	SAT
Active Rest	Resistance Training: Total Body	Active Rest	Resistance Training: Total Body	Active Rest	Resistance Training: Total Body	Cycling

Or this:

SUN	MON	TUE	WED	THU	FRI	SAT
Cycling	Active Rest	Resistance Training: Lower Body	Resistance Training: Upper Body	Active Rest	Resistance Training: Total Body	Active Rest

The point is, you can create just about any training schedule you want. It's plugging in the right workouts that makes or breaks it.

SEVEN-DAY SCHEDULE

Just for kicks, here's an example of a seven-day training program for someone committed to daily workouts:

SUN	MON	TUE	WED	THU	FRI	SAT
5k Walk with Dog	Resistance Training: Total Body	Cardio: Core Training*	Resistance Training: Total Body	Yoga	Resistance Training: Total Body	Abs, Arms & Ass Bootcamp*

These are specialty programs held at The Transformation Club®.

Find the schedule that works for you and get started. Be sure to remember the section on Minimum Effective Loading. You don't need to jump all-in all at once. Start with a schedule you can stick to—consistency is key!

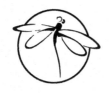

chapter 18

A FEW WORDS ABOUT WARMING UP

You might be tempted to skip the warm-up when you work out. After all, you only have so much time to exercise—*"Let's just get on with it already! I'm in a hurry!"*

But warming up is a critical component of your fitness routine and skipping it could have unpleasant and even dangerous results—muscle strain, injury, and pain.

Oh, and a proper warm-up will actually improve your workout performance!

THE WARM-UP: BASICS

A warm-up is a short workout period at the beginning of your exercise session. It is generally low intensity and prepares your body for the upcoming exertion.

The purpose of a traditional warm-up is to slightly increase your heart rate. This raises your core body temperature and increases the blood flow to your muscles. Cold muscles and other connective tissues do not stretch very easily. A warm-up session literally warms them up and relaxes them, making them more supple and ready to work.

Without a warm-up, you will be more susceptible to strained muscles, cramps, and injury. Ultimately, these effects could keep you from exercising for an extended period of time as you recover, which is not conducive to the healthy lifestyle you desire.

It takes about three minutes for your body to realize that it needs to move more blood to your muscles, so the ideal warm-up time is between five and ten minutes.

There is no set prescription for what your warm-up should consist of. You can choose a set of preparatory exercises (such as squats, lunges, toe touches, etc.), or you can do a light intensity version of your upcoming workout (a brisk walk to prepare for a run, for example, or lifting light weights before increasing the load).

THE WARM-UP: ADVANCED STRATEGY

For long-term health and fitness combined with your weight-loss training efforts, it's imperative to understand that a proper warm-up is about more than just warming up the body. It's about preparing the body for an all-out training assault that's going to boost your metabolism through the roof.

Look at the warm-up as a preparation phase for the workout to follow. Through research and practical experience, we've determined that best results are typically seen when a workout prep routine incorporates three key components:

1. Tissue quality

2. Corrective exercise

3. Mobility and activation

Tissue Quality

Almost all chronic joint pain or overuse injuries are caused by tightness and restrictions in the muscles above and below the joint in question.

In other words, it's not about pain site—it's about *pain source!*

Knee pain is often caused by restrictions in the tissue of your calves and front/inner/outer thighs. Back pain is often caused by restrictions in your glutes and hamstrings. Shoulder pain is often caused by restrictions in your thoracic spine (T-Spine), chest, and lats.

Tissue quality describes the general health of your muscles and the interconnected web of fascia that surrounds them all. Over time, we develop scar tissue, adhesions, knots, and trigger points due to high-intensity training, overuse, and/or extended periods of sitting.

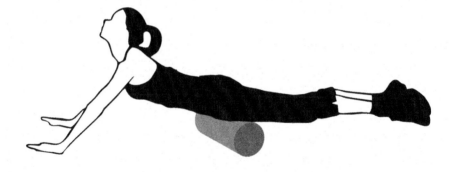

The best way to address this is to self-massage sore, tight, and restricted muscle groups of the body to regenerate tissue both pre- and post-workout to promote injury reduction and allow for a smoother, more productive workout.

In addition, self-massage before stretching allows for a better, more complete stretch by smoothing out the knots. You should always precede flexibility work with tissue quality for best results.

Self-massage is one of those counterintuitive things whereby you are actually actively searching for pain. In fact, it's the only time to ever do so when it comes to proper training. The best analogy I can give you is this:

If it hurts that much when you put pressure on your muscles, just imagine how bad your joints must feel!

Here is an example of 16-exercise 30:10 Tissue Quality Circuit, where we perform self-massage techniques using a ball and foam roller:

1. Chest/Shoulder – L

2. Chest/Shoulder – R

3. Lat (arm pit) – L

4. Lat (arm pit) – R

5. Back/Spine

6. Inner Thigh – L

7. Inner Thigh – R

8. Quad (front of thigh) – L

9. Quad (front of thigh) – R

10. Side of Thigh – L

11. Side of Thigh – R

12. Glute (butt) – L

13. Glute (butt) – R

14. Hamstring (back of thigh) – L

15. Hamstring (back of thigh) – R

16. Back/Spine

> *To see a video of the Tissue Quality Circuit, visit www.TheTransformationClub.fitness/ TissueQualityCircuit.*

By the way, we highly recommend including regular therapeutic massage as part of your overall training program—even if you start with just one session every Recovery Week.

Corrective Exercise

We all have unique "issues" with our body mechanics and functional movement capabilities. For some, it's a lack of flexibility, while others there may be a balance or mobility issue. Perhaps there's an asymmetry—one side is significantly "stronger" than the other leading to muscular imbalances, postural distortions, and overcompensation injuries.

To determine these "dysfunctions" we perform the Functional Movement Screen (FMS) on our members and ourselves.

The FMS is a ranking and grading system that documents movement patterns that are key to normal function. By screening these patterns, the FMS readily identifies functional limitations and asymmetries. These are issues that can reduce the effects of functional training and physical conditioning and distort body awareness. The FMS generates a score, which is used to target problems and track progress. This scoring system is directly linked to the most beneficial corrective exercises to restore mechanically sound movement patterns. Exercise professionals monitor the FMS score to track progress and to identify those exercises that will be most effective to restore proper movement and build strength in each individual.[43] So, in a nutshell, FMS is designed to:

43   www.functionalmovement.com

- identify functional limitations and asymmetries which have been linked to increased injury risk

- provide exercises to restore proper movement, and build stability, mobility, and strength in each individual

You can learn more about the FMS at www.functionalmovement.com.

Mobility & Activation

More than just a typical warm-up, a mobility and activation circuit truly prepares your body for a maximum performance workout.

Mobility describes the ability of a joint, or a series of joints, to move through an ideal range of motion. Though mobility relies on flexibility, it requires additional strength, stability, and a neuromuscular control component to allow for proper movement. Activation is often paired with mobility because many mobility exercises activate key, and often dormant, pillar stabilizers in your hips, core, and shoulders.

Here's an example of a mobility and activation routine:

1. Crocodile Breathing

2. Front Pillar

3. Cat-Cow

4. Bird Dog – L

5. Bird Dog – R

6. Downward Dogs

7. Slow Mountain Climber – L

8. Slow Mountain Climber – R

9. Split Squat or Reverse Lunge – L

10. Split Squat or Reverse Lunge – R

11. Lateral Squat or Lateral Lunge – L

12. Lateral Squat or Lateral Lunge – R

13. Hip Hinges

14. Hip Hinge to Push-up Walkout

15. Squats

16. Jumping Jacks

As you can see, a warm-up is much more than just a warm-up when you're training smarter for long-term health, fitness, and fat-loss goals.

To see a video of the mobility and activation circuit, visit www.TheTransformationClub.fitness/MobilityActivationCircuit.

chapter 19

HOW TO CHOOSE THE BEST EXERCISES FOR YOU

This is a very important concept to understand before beginning any training program. This is an article written by Justin that we felt compelled to share here.

There are countless exercises that you can perform with all kinds of equipment. The list is almost endless. There are hundreds, maybe thousands if you consider variations, that you can do with just your body weight alone!

So, how on earth do you determine what is the best exercise for a given goal, and better yet, is it the best one for *you*?

The truth is, you don't. Well, sort of . . .

Let me try to make some sense of this so you've got a solid takeaway by the end of this article.

CHOOSING THE BEST EXERCISES

First and foremost, can you really determine what is the *best* exercise for a given goal?

Personally, I don't think so. I mean, let's say we wanted to be really specific about our goal here—*a great butt!* After all, who doesn't want a *kickass backside*?

I'm also going with this example because, while a nice butt is good to look at, a strong functional set of glute muscles is critical to good physical health. Weak glutes are a common factor in knee and low-back pain.

We're going to attack this from a muscle development/shaping point of view. Remember, you *cannot* spot reduce (remove fat from an area by doing a specific exercise for that area). That'd be like chewing gum to slim down your face. It just doesn't happen.

Let's assume we're doing everything else right (nutrition, stress management, sleep, overall activity, etc.) to shed unwanted flab from down under and now we just want to give that booty some nice *pop*.

There's a whole slew of exercises that work the butt, from bridge variations, hinging exercises, split squat variations, step-up variations, and so on.

Can anyone really say which one is best? Well, the best one is probably the one you're *not* doing.

In other words, over time your body adapts to the stimulus you give it based on the old FITT principle—Frequency, Intensity, Time, Type. We won't get into that here, but just understand that you can't keep doing the same thing over and over expecting a different result—Einstein said that was the definition of insanity.

Let's talk about how *you* should choose exercises.

Keeping with our building a beautiful butt theme, it's easy to make the mistake of just picking a few of the proven butt builders, spreading them throughout your weekly training program and going from there. Hit them for a few weeks and then change up, right?

Wrong!

Here's the problem. We still haven't gotten down to *you.*

First and foremost, we should take a look at your function.

We have to look beyond your ability to perform an exercise, even if you can do it with decent form. Instead, we have to look at how functional you are in the overall movement pattern. We've already broken down Functional Movement Screening (FMS) for you.

In order to better understand the FMS, let's take a look at some of the "rules" the system is based on:

- Pain should not be present while performing basic body-weight movement patterns. If there is pain associated with these basic movement patterns, then they will be compromised and substantially increase the likelihood for developing further injury to the site of pain. Also, this could lead to a secondary injury from the body compensating to avoid the pain or restricted movement.

- Having multiple limitations within several basic movement patterns, *even if they're pain free,* can create compensations and general weaknesses that may lead to a greater likelihood of injury.

- Basic unilateral movement patterns should be symmetrical on both right and left sides of the body.

- Fundamental and basic movement patterning should precede performance related activities.

  □ Basic before complex, stable before unstable.

Using the Functional Movement Screening, we are able to establish a solid baseline to help manage and prevent injury to the musculoskeletal system. Plus, by establishing a baseline scoring criteria, we will be able to monitor and track progress to ensure that the right exercises are being implemented.

REAL-LIFE EXAMPLE—BACK TO THE BEAUTIFUL BUTT

Let's try to put all that into some real-life examples.

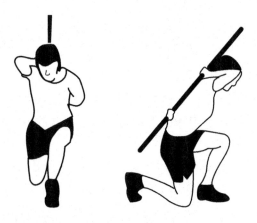

You go through the FMS and discover that you have a dysfunctional in-line lunge pattern.

Now, given this particular dysfunction, we know that it's in your best interest to avoid the following exercises:

- sagittal lunge variations (split squats, reverse lunges, forward lunges)

- running

So given our goal of building a beautiful backside we know right off the bat what exercises *not* to do. Fortunately, there are still many exercises to choose from to blast your butt.

Oh, and knowing that you have this dysfunction, we can also provide a list of exercises known to correct the dysfunction.

But, *what if lunges don't hurt?*

I can't tell you how many times I've been asked that one . . .

Remember, the FMS "rules"? Review this one:

- Having multiple limitations within several basic movement patterns, *even if they're pain free,* can create compensations and general weaknesses that may lead to a greater likelihood of injury.

This is something that comes up frequently with clients. They want to work hard, but sometimes you have to *pull on the reins* a bit to protect them from themselves. By ignoring your movement dysfunction, you're putting yourself at risk for injury, and for what? So you can do a lunge (in this example)—*are you trying to be a great lunger or have a great ass?*

If it's the ass you're after, then wouldn't it make more sense to choose another exercise that works the same muscles but doesn't have the risk and fix the dysfunction so the exercise no longer poses a risk?

Oh, and one more thing to consider: there's a pretty good chance that if you're doing the movement with a dysfunction you're not actually working the targeted muscles the way you want to. Your compensated movement pattern has to call upon other muscles to help out. For example, when you lunge with a dysfunctional in-line lunge movement pattern you tend to use your quads more—*you're not even working your glutes!*

BUTT-BLASTING AND ASS-SAVING ROUTINE

Let me give you an example of a workout (pretending you have in-line lunge dysfunction) that will actually work your glutes well and save you from yourself.

NOTE: *This is not a total body routine but simply an example of a series of exercise you could perform in a workout.*

Part 1: Fixing the Dysfunction

Now, the truth is there could be a variety of things causing the dysfunction, but I'll base this on the common things that I see:

Tissue Quality Work

Softball glutes	30–60 seconds each
Foam roll quads	30–60 seconds each
Foam roll IT bands	30–60 seconds each

Corrective Work

Side-lying clamshells	20 reps each
Cook hip lifts	10–15 reps each
Half kneeling hip flexors	10 reps each

Flexibility Work

Z-sits	30–60 seconds each
Half kneeling quad stretch	30–60 seconds each
Ankle mobilization drills	30–60 seconds each

Part 2: Kicking Ass

Here is just one of a bazillion examples of a strength workout you could do. I kept it basic and *old-school* using straight sets. A long-term program should manipulate exercise selection, sets, reps, tempo, combinations, etc.

Strength Work

Hip bridge variation	2 x 20
Romanian deadlifts	3 x 8 (assuming *no* active straight leg dysfunction)
Goblet squats	3 x 8 (assuming *no* deep squat dysfunction)
Hip thruster variation	2 x 12

OTHER DYSFUNCTIONAL CONSIDERATIONS

The Functional Movement Screen assesses *seven* key movement patterns:

1. Active straight leg raise

2. Shoulder mobility

3. Rotary stability

4. Torso stability push-up

5. In-line lunge

6. Hurdle step

7. Deep squat

My friends Steve Long and Jared Woolever, creators of www. SmartGroupTraining.com, created this chart to guide you on which exercises to avoid with each dysfunction:

SMART GROUP TRAINING RED LIGHTS

Active Straight Leg Raise	Shoulder Mobility	Rotary Stability	Torso Stability Push Up	In-Line Lounge	Hurdle Stop	Deep Squat
– Deadlifting – Hip Dominant Exercises • Swings • Cleans • Snatches – Running	– Overhead Pressing – Open Chain Horizontal Pressing • Bench Press • DB Bench • Plate Press – Get ups	– Power • Olympic Lifting • Cleans • Snatches • Push press • Swings – Running	– Push Up (from the floor or a more advanced progression)	– Lunges – Running	– Running – Jumping	– Resisted/ Weight Squatting – Jumping

Red Lights: Exercises guaranteed to cause more harm than good with a 1, asymmetrical 1, or pain in a particular movement pattern

Keep this in mind—It's not about punishing you and taking your favorite exercises away from you. It's about selecting the right exercises for you, fixing the dysfunction, and putting those exercises back into your program.

KNOW BETTER—DO BETTER

Janell has a saying that goes something like this, "Now that you know better, it's up to you to do better."

In other words, you can keep doing what you're doing—hoping for the best and ignoring the worst—*or* you can work with a trained professional (like me) who is first and foremost concerned with your long-term results.

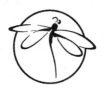

chapter 20

YOUR TRANSFORMATION WORKOUT PROGRAM

After what's been covered up to this point in the training program section of this book, it should go without saying that there is not one perfect transformation workout program; there are simply good places to start.

We provide our members with a new workout program every mesocycle, so we obviously can't say, "Here's the workout—go!" On the flip side, we can't fill this book with years' worth of programs.

Instead, we're going to give you a workout program that we really like and know will work wonders for you as you start your transformation. Then, if you'd like to get continuous programming and/or coaching, you can explore the options at www.TheTransformationClub. fitness.

RESISTANCE TRAINING PROGRAM

For the resistance training program, we're going to give you two training style options:

1. Metabolic Resistance Training, like you would see in our Group Personal Training program

2. Alternating Set Method with a HIIT finisher, like you might see in our Personal Training program

For the MRT workout, we provided a total body workout version to be performed on nonconsecutive days and a two-day split routine that gives you the option to work out two days in a row if you want/have to.

MRT Program

Directions: You will alternate between thirty seconds of maximum work and fifteen seconds of rest for each exercise in the following six-exercise circuit. You will then take a sixty-second rest before repeating the circuit. Perform two to six times, depending on your current fitness level and the time you have available.

Total Body Routine

STATION #	WORKOUT A	WORKOUT B	WORKOUT C
1	Single-Leg RDLs	Swings	Hip Thrusts
2	Push-Ups	Overhead Press	Chest Press
3	Front Squats	Alternating Reverse Lunges	Lateral Lunges
4	Pulldowns	Low Rows	High Rows
5	Bodysaw	Chops	Side Pillar
6	Slams	Squat Jumps	Jumping Jacks

Split Routine

STATION #	WORKOUT A	WORKOUT B
1	Swings	Squats
2	Pulldowns	Chest Press
3	Hip Thrusts	Alternating Lunges
4	Rows	Overhead Press
5	Hammer Curls	Triceps Extensions
6	Mountain Climbers	Burpees

Alternating Set Method

Directions: Perform Exercise A followed by the designated rest period. Then perform Exercise B followed by the designated rest period. Repeat for the total number of sets before moving to the next pair of exercises.

WORKOUT A	WORKOUT B	SETS X REPS	REST PERIOD
1A) Romanian Deadlifts	1A) Squats	2–4 x 8–10	60 seconds
1B) Push-Ups	1B) Rows	2–4 x 8–10	60 seconds
2A) Hip Thrusts	2A) Lunges	2–3 x 10–12	45 seconds
2B) Overhead Presses	2B) Pulldowns	2–3 x 10–12	45 seconds
3A) Triceps Extensions	3A) Hammer Curls	2–3 x 12–15	30 seconds
3B) Alternating Dead Bugs	3B) Ab Wheel Rollouts	2–3 x 12–16	30 seconds
4) Mountain Climbers	4) Burpees	6 x 30 seconds	30 seconds

CARDIO TRAINING PROGRAM

If your morning resting heart rate is above seventy beats per minute, choose a lower intensity form of cardio to improve your aerobic base. Just be cautious of the duration and the pounding on your joints. Start with twenty to thirty minutes of low-impact exercise like biking, brisk walking, swimming, rowing, etc.

If you're morning resting heart rate is below seventy beats per minute, bring on the HIIT. However, that doesn't mean you have to *kill it!*

For the HIIT cardio training program, we're going to give you two options:

1. Alactic-aerobic intervals—follow this program if you're a beginner and/or are new to HIIT cardio.

2. Glycolytic intervals—follow this program if you're a more advanced trainee and have recent experience with HIIT cardio.

Feel free to choose any cardio/conditioning exercise you enjoy that you're able to generate a lot of intensity. Examples include bike sprints, running sprints, medicine ball slams, battling rope waves, mountain climbers, burpees, shadow boxing, shuffles, jumping rope, jumping jacks, rowing machine, etc.

The idea is to go *all-out* for the time that you're "on." Then move at a comfortable recovery pace for the "off" period. For example, sprint for the "on" and walk for the "off."

Perform your HIIT cardio workouts one to two times per week on nonconsecutive days, preferably on days you're not performing resistance training.

WEEK	ALACTIC-AEROBIC INTERVALS	GLYCOLYTIC INTERVALS
1	10 seconds on, 50 seconds off 6 rounds	30 seconds on, 90 seconds off 5 rounds
2	10 seconds on, 50 seconds off 8 rounds	30 seconds on, 90 seconds off 6 rounds
3	10 seconds on, 50 seconds off 10 rounds	30 seconds on, 90 seconds off 7 rounds
4	10 seconds on, 50 seconds off 12 rounds	30 seconds on, 90 seconds off 8 rounds
5	10 seconds on, 50 seconds off 15 rounds	30 seconds on, 90 seconds off 9 rounds
6	10 seconds on, 50 seconds off 15 rounds	30 seconds on, 90 seconds off 10 rounds

NOTE: *If you find your heart rate settling in to "resting level" and you feel ready to go before your rest period complete, shorten your rest periods.*

BONUS CARDIO: We've seen tremendous benefit from following up your HIIT session with twenty to thirty minutes of low- to moderate-intensity steady-state cardio. Some call it "stubborn fat" cardio because it takes advantage of the hormonal shift that occurs after HIIT and has been shown to aid in burning fat, especially in the "stubborn" areas like your hips, belly, and thighs.

DON'T FORGET THE COOLDOWN

Too many people bolt at the end of their workout because they think the important work is done. We disagree. Cooling down after your workout is definitely important.

According to the National Academy of Sports Medicine (NASM), a cool-down provides the body with a smooth transition from exercise back to a steady state of rest.

"The overarching goal of a cool-down," NASM says, *"is to reduce heart and breathing rates, gradually cool body temperature, return muscles to their optimal length-tension relationships, prevent venous pooling of blood in the lower extremities, which may cause dizziness or possible fainting, and restore physiologic systems close to baseline."*[44]

The proposed benefits of a cooldown are:

- reduce heart and breathing rates

- gradually cool body temperature

- return muscles to their optimal length-tension relationships

- prevent venous pooling of blood in the lower extremities

- restore physiologic systems close to baseline

This is also a really great time to work on your flexibility since your muscles are quite warm. Entire books have been written about flexibility so we'll just close this section with the cooldown/flexibility routine we perform at the end of our Group Personal Training workouts at The Transformation Club®:

1. ½ Kneeling Hip Flexor/Quad Stretch – L

2. ½ Kneeling Hip Flexor/Quad Stretch – R

3. Cat/Cow

4. Child's Pose

5. Z Sit – L

6. Z Sit – R

7. Seated Hamstring Stretch – L

8. Seated Hamstring Stretch – R

---

44   www.NASM.org

9. Open Book – L

10. Open Book – R

11. Supine Breathing

Perform each exercise/stretch for thirty seconds. Perform silent breathing for as long as you like.

To see a video of the Flexibility circuit, visit www.TheTransformationClub.fitness/ FlexibilityCircuit.

PART 4

THE LIFESTYLE PROGRAM

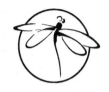

chapter 21

THE MANY FACES OF STRESS

Here is the thing about stress: you could be eating the most "perfect" supportive nutrition plan, but if your body is under too much stress, you will not see the results that you are looking for.

"Stress is any influence, internal or external, that causes or leads to malfunction."

"Stress is often well hidden and may involve several layers of investigation."

—Reed Davis

Stress is natural, but it's the way that we perceive and handle it that is important. While a little bit of stress sharpens our attention, too much stress and anxiety are like a "parking brake" on our performance. There is a zone of "optimal stress." If you are like most people in our overstressed, fast-paced modern world, then you probably need to calm down rather than rev up.

Some stress can be good. Good stress helps you learn, grow, and get stronger. Exercise can be a form of good stress. You feel a little uncomfortable but then you feel good, and it lasts for a short time period.

 ## EFFECTS OF STRESS

- Fifty percent of all illnesses are caused by stress.

- Seventy to eighty percent of visits to a doctor are related to stress and stress-related factors.[45]

Too much stress can have disastrous effects on your attitude, posture, and body's hormone levels. Stress is not just physical, mental, and emotional. Stress can be chemical and/or functional. Toxins from personal care products, cleaning products, and food also put tremendous amounts of stress on our bodies.

When your body reacts to stress, the stress hormone, cortisol, is usually involved. Anything that elevates cortisol (stress, parasitic infection, food sensitivities, inflammation, etc.) will elevate blood sugar, therefore elevating insulin as well. Remember, insulin is our fat storage hormone. Again, you could have the "perfect" supportive nutrition plan and exercise program, but if cortisol is chronically elevated, you are most likely increasing your blood sugar from the inside.

Improper nutrition from excess sugar and/or carbohydrates, excessively large meals can excessively elevate blood sugar levels. When blood sugar spikes fast and high, it will crash very low. Our body views this as a stressful event and, therefore, will kick out cortisol. It

---

45   Functional Diagnostic Nutrition, "Stress Reduction," *Functional Diagnostic Nutrition* (blog), http://bonesandhormones.com/fdn/stress-reduction/.

is a vicious cycle between cortisol, blood sugar, and insulin. It is very important to eat meals and food that help to keep our blood sugar stable throughout the day. This will decrease the stress our body is under.

> **NOTE:** *Hormones, not calories, control our metabolism and, therefore, control our weight.*

Long-term psychological stress increases the hormones and cell-signaling molecules that make you fatter, sicker, and weaker, as well as inhibits the hormones and cell-signaling molecules that make you leaner, healthier, and stronger.

Stress that includes dwelling on negative thoughts can literally cause brain damage. Cortisol (our stress hormone) released in stressful situations damages the hippocampus, which helps us learn and form memories. Adrenaline dumps sugar into our bloodstream and inflammatory chemicals start oxidizing brain plaques, which contributes to neurodegenerative diseases, such as Alzheimer's.

Impact of Dysregulated Stress Hormones

The impact of dysregulated (not regulated normally) stress hormones can include:

- headaches, dizziness, ADD/ADHD, anxiety, irritability and anger, panic disorder
- grinding teeth and tension in the jaw
- breakdown of lean muscle tissue
- increased risk for type 2 diabetes
- weight gain and obesity
- food cravings

241

- decreased DHEA (anti-aging hormone)

- increased blood sugar

- decreased production of thyroid gland

- increased blood pressure

- increased cholesterol and triglycerides

- decreased sex drive

- sleep disturbances

- decreased serotonin and melatonin

- depressed immune system

Stress also impacts your digestive system by decreasing enzymes, bacteria, and acids required for proper digestion, absorption, and metabolism. It also contributes to "leaky gut," which can cause weight gain, hormone imbalance, GI symptoms such as bloating and gas, and autoimmune conditions.

The bottom line is that stress affects the entire body and can cause many other problems, such as insomnia, emotional and behavioral problems, immune system dysfunction, asthma, ulcers, lack of energy, depression, nervousness, paranoia, etc.

MANAGE YOUR STRESS, MANAGE YOUR BLOOD SUGAR

Dysregulated blood sugar can be a major internal stressor on the body because of its relationship to cortisol. When your sympathetic nervous system is active and your body is in "flight or fight," your blood sugar increases. A significant increase in blood sugar causes an increase in insulin, which then causes an increase in cortisol, which causes an increase in blood sugar. And around and around it goes.

Stress increases cortisol, increases insulin, inhibits weight loss, and increases belly fat. Belly fat is always a cortisol and/or blood sugar issue.

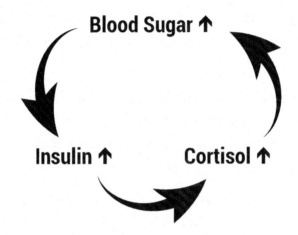

Enter the cycle in one of two ways.

- **Improper nutrition.** Excess sugar and/or carbohydrates, excessively large meals, or glycemically (*glycemic index is how quickly a food will increase your blood sugar*) imbalanced meals can excessively elevate blood sugar levels.

- **Can start with cortisol.** Anything that elevates cortisol (*stress, parasitic infection, food allergies, inflammation, etc.*) will elevate blood sugar, therefore insulin as well. You could have the perfect supportive nutrition plan and exercise program, but if cortisol is elevated, you are most likely increasing blood sugar from the inside.

NUTRITIONAL HABITS TO DECREASE STRESS

- **Avoid low blood sugar by avoiding high blood sugar**. The faster your blood sugar rises, the faster it will come down.

- **Choose foods that nourish your body rather than make it work harder**. Pesticides, herbicides, artificial ingredients, flavors, and preservatives cause the body to work harder to remove them.

- **Drink more water**. Dehydration has been shown to increase cortisol levels.

- **Increase anti-inflammatory omega-3 fatty acids**. Wild salmon and golden ground flax seeds can reduce inflammation.

- **Increase antioxidants**. Vegetables and fruits provide additional defense against stress. Aim for six to eight servings of non-starchy vegetables each day with a 3:1 ratio of vegetables to fruit servings.

- **Avoid processed and high-carbohydrate foods**.

- **Eat organic produce, pasture-raised, grass-fed meat whenever possible.**

- **Eat real food.**

You may also want to get a glucometer and test your blood sugar. It can provide you with valuable information. Test first thing in the morning, right before lunch, right before dinner, and before bed.

Ideally your blood sugar would be between eighty and ninety each time. *This may vary slightly for each individual.* If you are consistently over ninety when testing blood sugar, look at reducing carbohydrates and/or stress. If you are below eighty, add a small of carbohydrate and see how you feel. Testing blood sugar can be very beneficial information for what types of carbohydrates to eat and when.

If you decide to measure blood sugar, do it for two weeks. During that time keep track of what and how much you are eating at each meal. This will give you the information you need to make adjustments. This was very eye opening for us when we did it a few years ago. Periodically we will measure our blood sugar for a few days to see what is going on. **Keep in mind, it's simply information.**

Take Time to Relax

It's not sexy, it's not a quick fix, but taking time to relax each day *will* move you closer to your health and fitness goals. Relaxation can improve our overall outlook on life, our health, and our performance. It can also help you to get a good night's sleep.

Stress and sleep contain zero calories, and can have a big impact on our metabolism, health, and ability to lose and/or maintain weight.

When you are relaxed and less stressed, you are much more likely to make thoughtful choices, understand and remember all of the things you are learning, and perform better during workouts. Not only will relaxation help you to make more thoughtful choices, but you will also be more likely to view mistakes as learning experiences rather than as failures. In the long run, this will mean a leaner, healthier, and stronger body.

Here is the good news: you don't have to wait around for positive thoughts and feelings to appear; you can create them. You can also create a relaxed state of mind by training your body and mind. Just like pretty much anything else, relaxation is a habit. With practice, you can change your physiological and physical response.

Breathing

Some research says that anxiety and stress are related to low oxygen levels and high carbon dioxide levels. When we are stressed, we tend to breathe shallowly, like a fish out of water gasping for air! By changing our breathing, we can change our mental state.

For most people the word meditation is hard or boring. Even if you think you are doing it wrong and are the worst meditator in the world, we encourage you to try it for just three to five minutes.

Regular meditation:

- lowers blood pressure

- lowers heart rate

- lowers stress hormones

- lowers inflammation

- boosts immune system

- improves focus and mental clarity

- improves mood

- improves sleep

 MEDITATION BASICS

- Find a comfortable, quiet, private place.

- Sit or lie down, whatever seems most comfortable.

- Set a timer for three, five, or ten minutes.

- Close your eyes.

- Focus on your breath. You don't need to breathe in any special way. Just breathe and notice what it feels like. Observe how the air moves in and out.

- Let your thoughts drift in and out.

- Observe only; let go of any and all judgment.

- Keep coming back to your breath. You may want to try a mantra such as, "this moment." On your inhale you say to yourself "this" and on your exhale "moment." That way, when your mind wanders, you can keep coming back to your mantra.

NOTE: We both use the Headspace app and that works well for us.

POSITIVE SELF-TALK

Each and every day you have multiple conversations with yourself inside of your head. Your brain is always chatting away with itself, whether it's in words, images, or feelings. Most of the time, you simply aren't aware of it.

Are the stories and conversations you have with yourself impacting your health and well-being?

Our guess is the conversation you have with yourself isn't the nicest. Think about some of the stories, thoughts, and what you say inside your head to yourself each day. We bet you would never say the things you say to yourself to your best friend!

Research shows that self-talk (a.k.a. our inner conversations) has measurable effects on your body. Negative self-talk and negative social judgment (a.k.a. self-criticism) is often physiologically worse than physical stress. Every time you criticize yourself, you create a "real" bully that actually physically harms you. Being mean to yourself can be worse, physiologically speaking, than a hurricane.

Self-criticism and negative self-talk can have a negative impact on how you look, feel, and perform. Trust me when we say that you won't get more fit or any leaner from beating yourself up mentally.

Here is the good news. If you are prone to negative self-talk, *you can change.* Your brain is highly moldable, which means that all you have to do is put down some new brain pathways. Self-talk is a habit, just like eating vegetables, and habits can change.

Self-talk has physiological effects, but this works both ways. Negative self-talk has negative effects. Positive self-talk has positive effects. Why not make your brain work for you instead of against you? Start noticing and naming any negative thoughts and self-talk you have about your health, nutrition, and fitness. It may sound like this:

- *This is hard. I should quit.*

- *I'm never going to reach my goals.*

- *I don't know why I thought I could do this.*

- *I ate too much at lunch. I'm such a failure. I might as well keep on eating.*

Positive self-talk should feel real. You want to believe it. Start by listing some things that you truly feel good about, and/or things that you've been successful with. For example:

- I ate *x* serving of vegetables yesterday.

- I handled [insert challenge with food] better than I would have in the past.

- I tried *x* food for the first time and liked it!

Write out your list and keep it handy. Add to it as things come to you. What you will notice is as you start looking for the positives that you will see them more often. Once a day or several times per week, practice some positive self-talk. Pick one or two items from your list and sit with them. Really pay attention to how it makes you feel good, how accomplished you feel. Remind yourself of that great moment and make it as real as possible in your head.

Focus on what you are doing well, create vivid images of positive experiences, and work on doing more of that!

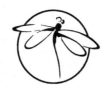

chapter 22

YOUR SELF-CARE TOOLBOX

Self-care is not selfish!

Previously we talked a bit about self-care, but we feel that it is so important that we are revisiting it here!

If you have ever flown on an airplane, you know the drill with the oxygen masks: put on your own oxygen mask first before assisting others. Yet in our everyday lives, how often are we putting everyone and everything before ourselves? If you try to be everything to everyone else without caring for yourself, you eventually run out of gas or become ill. And then you aren't much good to anyone.

If you don't care for yourself, how can you be the best spouse, mother/father, friend, coworker, etc.?

We all have physical, mental, and emotional demands being put on us each and every day. Whether it's caring for others, our careers, or simply tending to day-to-day life activities, we can feel our stress level skyrocket and be left feeling drained. But if we don't take care of ourselves, *how can we help others?*

Often self-care is viewed as selfish, and that is the furthest thing from the truth! *What good are you to other people if you are sick or burned out?* Think of self-care practices as the "anchors" that let you weather the storms, rather than self-indulgences.

Every time you say yes to something, you are saying no to something else. For years, Janell said yes to everyone but herself. She just could not say no and set healthy boundaries for herself. It wasn't until she was suffering from stage-3 adrenal fatigue that she finally had to start saying yes to herself. Janell had to start putting her self-care at the top of the list instead of only caring for herself when there was time, which most of the time never happened. If she didn't, she was headed down a path of chronic fatigue, carrying excess weight, and eventually more serious health conditions.

Managing your stress is crucial to your overall health and well-being. Over the course of many years, Janell identified the behaviors and actions that were moving her closer to optimal health and well-being and the ones that weren't. She began prioritizing and making the time for taking care of herself. Instead of watching TV during the week, she started spending more time in the kitchen preparing whole unprocessed foods. She stepped outside of her comfort zone and starting attending a weekly yoga class. And positive behaviors and actions stemmed from there.

STRESS-MANAGEMENT TOOLS

Here are some tools to help you manage stress:

- managing your time

- engaging the parasympathetic nervous system

- taking a detox bath

- exercise

- changing your perception
- focusing on a positive attitude
- yoga
- meditation
- massage
- reading
- spending time with pets
- laughing
- doing what you enjoy
- gratitude journal
- high-quality supportive nutrition
- supplements
- spending time with those you love
- getting in nature
- belly breath
- prioritizing sleep

Everyone's self-care toolbox is going to look different. You may have three things that you do to practice self-care or you may have ten. There is not a right or wrong when it comes to self-care. Self-care is simply behaviors and/or actions that help you to destress and move you toward more optimal health and well-being.

The important thing is that self-care becomes part of your daily routine. Some days you may devote five minutes to deep breathing or being in nature. And other days may be full of self-care: a morning yoga class, a nutrient-dense lunch with friends, an afternoon walk in nature, and reading a great book before bed. Self-care may ebb and flow as things change in your life. The key is to be aware of how you can best care for yourself no matter what your situations or circumstances.

OPTIMIZE SLEEP

Sleep restores everything in our bodies: our immune, nervous, skeletal, hormonal, and muscular systems.

Sleep helps regulate our metabolism, including blood sugar and insulin levels. Eventually, chronically inadequate sleep can actually make us gain body fat and become diabetic. Sleep helps us make and recall memories. We think, learn, and make decisions better when we are well rested.

Recent research shows that while different people function best with different amounts of sleep each night, fewer than 2 percent of people thrive with fewer than seven hours per night. Missing sleep messes with our metabolism. Because sleep helps regulate our blood sugar, lack of sleep can actually cause or worsen insulin resistance and type 2 diabetes, even in healthy people. Less sleep also means more cravings the following day. The less you sleep, the more likely you are to gain weight, snack excessively, or have one of a host of mood disorders.

Sleep and stress have zero calories and you can't eat them, but they dramatically impact what you choose to eat, how much of it you eat, and whether it will be burned or stored once you eat it."

—Jade Teta

How Light Affects Our Sleep

Our circadian rhythm is our internally driven, twenty-four-hour *"around the day"* that automatically cues physical, mental, and behavioral processes, including sleeping and waking that keep our body in balance. While our circadian rhythm is built in and self-sustained, it's also affected by external environmental cues, like daylight and darkness.

Several factors control our circadian rhythm, but the biggest is our exposure to light. Before electricity, we would generally go to bed when the sun went down (or close to it) and get up when the sun came up (or close to it). These natural light/dark cycles drove our circadian rhythms. And since the sun was so regular, so were our sleep schedules.

Fast-forward to today, and few of us follow a sun-based sleep schedule any longer. Other sources of artificial light now interfere with our internal body clocks. Daytime light is wonderful; it wakes us up and regulates us. Aim to get as much as possible. Night-time light is not so great; it messes with our body clock, making it harder to fall asleep and/or stay asleep. Reduce or eliminate it as much as you can.

Tips for reducing light exposure:

- Avoid electronic screens several hours before bed. If you must be on your computer, dim the brightness.

- Use a dim alarm clock or one that gradually lights up in the morning.

- Get good darkening shades.

- Wear blue blocker glasses or amber goggles after dark that block blue light. This is the light that decreases our production of melatonin (sleep hormone).

You can't always determine how much or how well you will actually sleep. Whether it's kids, pets, shift work, hormonal issues, sleep apnea, or other factors playing a role. What you can do is take charge of your sleep routine and control your sleep behaviors, which will dramatically improve your chances of good, restful sleep.

Create a good sleep routine:

- Decide on a bedtime in advance, and start planning for it one to two hours ahead.

- Limit your caffeine to the morning with absolutely no caffeinated drinks after 2 p.m.

- One to two hours before bed, take out a piece of paper and do a "brain dump."

- Turn off all electronic screens (TV, computer, etc.) an hour before bed.

- Make yourself some decaf tea, listen to soft music, and read something light.

- Turn off all phones and gadgets and put them in another room.

- Set your bedroom temperature to sixty-seven to sixty-eight degrees Fahrenheit.

- Take an Epsom salt bath before bed.

- Dim the light; darken your bedroom.

- Try some white noise, like a humidifier.

- Focus on your behaviors rather than the outcomes.

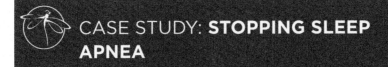

CASE STUDY: **STOPPING SLEEP APNEA**

When I came to Transformation Club, I had a very bad food habit and was overweight. More importantly, I had severe obstructive sleep apnea. Around nine months before joining the club, I removed my large tonsils with the hope that it would help control my apnea. My apnea episodes per hour went down from fifty-four to nine, but then due to me being over-weight, it again went up to the twenties within nine months. I was also borderline in cholesterol, and tri-glycerides were high. It was time to take a decision.

I had tried doing things by myself, even trying OTC detox pills, weight-control crap, etc., but no result. Joining the six-week challenge was a huge eye opener. Group Personal Training helped in staying motivated and focusing on making better choices. I had a great six-week challenge and lost over twenty-four pounds. But more importantly, I lost additional pounds after the challenge was over and have been making some better choices on food habits. It has helped a lot and improved my sleep quality. I also do not get frequent headaches and rarely feel fatigue. The great news was that I tested last week for my sleep apnea, and I don't have any at the moment. So it has gone down from the twenties to single digits without having to tamper with my body. The Eniva products have also been great!!

I still have a long way to go, as this is a lifestyle versus a one-time thing, and I will continue to monitor my apnea, but indeed the club has left a good impact on my life. My wife calls me a health fanatic at the moment.

—Biplap Mandal

chapter 23

MINDFUL EATING

How you eat can be just as important as what you eat—it can allow you to eat less overall but still leave you nutritionally, physically, emotionally, and mentally satisfied. Take a moment to think about how you feel when you eat slowly while sitting down with good company. Our guess is that feeling is very different than when you eat while driving, watching TV, or while standing at the kitchen counter.

We have all had those times when we ate a meal that left us bloated, regretful, or feeling like we hadn't eaten at all. It is likely that during that meal we didn't really taste our food, we ate very quickly, and our environment didn't support mindful and conscious eating.

What if you left the table feeling light, lean, full of energy, yet satisfied? Well you can, it's simple, but not easy and it's going to take a bit of practice. *Always, no matter the situation, eat slowly.* When people eat fast, they end up eating more. But even with more food, they don't feel satisfied. Five minutes later, they are looking for seconds or dessert. An hour later, they are looking for a snack.

Quite the opposite happens to those that eat slowly. Those individuals usually end up eating a lot less, yet they feel more satisfied. They also feel calmer and happier. They don't have to think about eating less, they just naturally do it.

Your brain doesn't get the full signal until about twenty minutes after you start eating. We would bet that most of your meals don't even last that long. The process of seeing your food, to the moment it hits your intestines, to your body making enzymes and hormones to digest the food and telling your brain that you have had enough, is *slow.*

But here is the great thing: your body knows how much it needs. Your job is to help it by eating slowly and mindfully. Eat slowly and then trust your body. Trust yourself to relearn what "full" actually feels like. This will take practice and then some more practice.

EAT TO 80 PERCENT FULL

Most people eat, or continue eating, regardless of whether or not their body actually needs the food. We often don't stop eating until the plate (or container) is empty.

Eating to 80 percent can help you to eat consciously, "tune in" to your body's true hunger and satiation signals, improve your digestion, and be a foundational practice you can always come back to.

However, it may give you an uneasy feeling to actually leave food on your plate and listen to the cues your body gives you when it has had enough food. Many people feel this way. "Wasting food" can feel bad. It can bring up the past or heavy emotions. It's important to recognize and work through these thoughts and feelings.

Unprocessed foods (such as fresh vegetables and fruits, animal proteins, and healthy fats) will help you feel full sooner and for longer. Processed foods mess with your body's natural signals, and you'll often never get to the 80 percent full point.

Start to practice stopping eating just a little sooner than you normally would or try using a smaller plate. Eating slowly will help you to do that. These two habits will take a lot of practice; the idea is to just do a little bit better today and then build from there.

 ## MINDFUL EATING EXERCISE

Over the course of this next week, set aside fifteen minutes with no interruptions or distractions to complete this mindful eating exercise. Before beginning the exercise, grab a handful of nuts or grapes or a few chunks of fresh fruit that you have available.

- **Set your nuts or fruit out in front of you and look at them.** Pick a piece up and look at it closely. Notice how each piece is different.

- **Sniff the food.** Does it have a smell? Can you identify the scent?

- **Pop the nut or grape into your mouth.** Roll it around a bit, feeling the texture.

- **Bite into it.** Notice what happens to your taste buds. Chew it slowly. Does the taste and texture change as you chew? Chew the piece of food fifteen times.

- Then swallow the piece of food and repeat with the remaining pieces.

You don't need to eat all of your meals this way. This exercise simply shows you how much more you can experience and enjoy your food when you slow down, pay attention, and eat mindfully.

TYPES OF HUNGER

Before you eat do you pause to ask yourself, *Am I physically hungry?* Or do you find yourself with food in hand, thinking, *I'm not even hungry right now!*

Physical Hunger

The feeling of hunger builds slowly and occurs several hours after a meal. A guideline would be roughly three to four hours. This may be how you feel after exercise or a long period of work, when your energy stores are depleted. Your stomach may begin to growl. If you don't eat soon, you might become tired and irritable, get a headache, or notice that it becomes harder to focus. This is your physiological need for nutrients and energy. After you eat, these hunger symptoms disappear almost instantly.

It's natural to feel physical hunger when your stomach is empty and your body is low on fuel. Physical hunger is a sign that your body is functioning well and responding to the right signals. When you feel physical hunger, feed your body.

Nutritional Hunger

Your body's cry for more nutrients. Eating a SAD full of processed and refined foods will leave you nutritionally bankrupt. These processed foods contain more than enough caloric energy, but they do nothing to satisfy your body's need for vitamins, minerals, phytonutrients, and enzymes. Even though your body is getting plenty of energy, it is still starving for nutrients. If your stomach feels full an hour or so after you have eaten, but you still can't focus or you feel tired, this is likely a sign of nutritional hunger.

Hormonal Hunger

This is a feeling of hunger that comes on suddenly. It often has nothing to do with mealtime. In fact, hormonal hunger can strike right after a big meal. This is also where that room for dessert comes from. Hormonal hunger can cause strong emotional cravings for specific foods, especially carbohydrates. It can often overpower even the strongest willpower. It can cause mood swings and low energy, and it creates a near continual desire to eat.

The "out of control" cravings that some people experience are not normal.

- How many times has your brain told you that you shouldn't eat something, but you can't say no and eat it anyway?

- Have you ever continued eating a meal because you think you're still hungry, and then feel uncomfortably full or even sick afterward?

- Have you ever felt cravings for more food and looked through the pantry for something to eat less than an hour after a big meal?

These feelings of hunger are not a lack of willpower: constant cravings and an appetite that is difficult to control are usually caused by eating the wrong foods. When you eat the foods your body is designed to eat, then your brain will stop signaling the need to eat.

Your cravings will be very minimal and likely disappear altogether. You will only feel hungry when your body truly has a need for fuel.

Hormonal hunger is the hunger responsible for emotional eating, binges, and irresistible cravings. It is primarily caused by eating too much sugar, grains, and starchy foods that put your hormones and blood sugar levels on a roller coaster. Using protein, healthy fats, and nonstarchy vegetables for the base of most meals and avoiding sugar, grains, and high starchy foods will retrain your brain to instruct your cells to burn fat as a fuel source.

Wanting to Eat vs. Needing to Eat

True hunger is general and nonspecific. It can be an empty, growling stomach, lightheadedness, or irritability. Hunger comes and goes, often gradually. Cravings, on the other hand, are *very* particular, usually for a certain kind of food. There are few signs of physical hunger, just a strong urge, sometimes felt in the back of the throat. A craving will come on suddenly and feels like an immediate compulsion.

Have you ever actually stopped before eating to check in with your body to see if you are actually hungry? Chances are if you practice some mindfulness around your eating you would discover that often we reach for food out of boredom, loneliness, anxiety, sadness, or stress. This is referred to as "emotional eating."

"Feeling" with our guts makes it easy to confuse emotions or other physical sensations with hunger.

Our brains have to coordinate input from multiple sources: our body fat, our gastrointestinal tract, our sensory organs, and other body systems. Emotions or physical sensations can feel like hunger because our brains also have to deal with our emotions, our physical feelings, our beliefs, and our thoughts.

Feel-Good Neurotransmitters

Serotonin and dopamine are neurotransmitters. Serotonin makes us feel groovy and relaxed. It also tells us to stop eating. Dopamine, in contrast, is our "reward" neurotransmitter. It gives us a "high." About 90 percent of our body's serotonin is actually in our GI tract. When we eat, we release serotonin and dopamine.

Individuals who struggle with overeating are often just trying to boost their levels of serotonin and dopamine. Eating carbohydrates (particularly simple sugars and starches) can help release serotonin, which soothes and relaxes us.

Dopamine is released in response to the "reward" of good-tasting food. Dopamine is involved in addictions such as gambling, compulsive shopping, and alcoholism. Dopamine is the chemical that encourages us to seek out the "hit" of a brief and intense thrill.

Eating can be a kind of "self-medication" that helps calm us or boost our mood. The movement of our jaw stimulates a nerve that helps release serotonin, as well. Food manufacturers understand the neurobiology and psychology and know that we are more likely to crave sugary, creamy, fatty, and salty foods. Such foods can become our "drugs" of choice because (just like other drugs) they make us feel better, at least for the short term. Unlike true hunger, it's hard to satisfy psychological hunger.

 TIPS TO HELP DEAL WITH CRAVINGS

- Understand that cravings are normal. They come and go.

- If the craving is minor, ignore it.

- If the craving is moderate, distract yourself.

- Keep a "craving diary." Write down the craving and when it happens. Write down what you are thinking at that time. Over time, look for patterns. Once you identify the pattern, you can disrupt it.

- Substitute something that gives you the same feeling. For example, take a detox bath when you are craving warmth and comfort. Go for a walk in nature when you crave a distraction. Drink water or herbal tea when you just want something to do with your mouth.

The good news is we can reduce cravings with supportive, smart food choices. Whole foods nourish us but don't give us the intense "hit" of processed foods. Serotonin and dopamine also depend to some degree on protein, fat, and micronutrient levels. If we eat plenty of protein and healthy fats along with a wide range of vitamins and minerals from whole foods, our brains are happy!

chapter 24

AN ATTITUDE OF GRATITUDE

Gratitude helps people feel more positive emotions, relish positive experiences, have better health, deal with adversity, and build strong relationships.[46]

When you set goals to improve your health, gain more energy, and/or lose weight, those goals often have to do with nutrition and exercise. And while these two aspects of living a healthy life are *very* important, what if we told you that appreciation and being thankful could increase your health and enhance your well-being?

Too often as a society we focus on the negative in situations and the people around us. We find ourselves blaming and playing the victim role. This doesn't serve us and can stick us into a negative, depressed-like mind-set.

46   Harvard Mental Health, "In Praise of Gratitude," *Harvard Health Publications* (blog), November 2011, www.health.harvard.edu/newsletter_article/in-praise-of-gratitude.

HOW PRACTICING GRATITUDE CAN IMPROVE YOUR HEALTH

There is an intimate relationship between thoughts, moods, brain chemistry, endocrine function, and the other physiological systems in your body. What this means is that what you think about has a direct impact on how you feel both physically and emotionally.

If you increase the amount of positive thoughts you have each day, you increase your overall sense of well-being as well as your physical health. Those who regularly practice gratitude report: *exercising more regularly, having fewer physical symptoms, sleeping better, having a stronger immune system, feeling more alive, and better resilience as it relates to stress.* But the benefits of practicing gratitude can be endless. *Psychology Today* reported that individuals that wrote down what they are grateful for before retiring for the night fell asleep faster and stayed asleep longer.[47]

Expressing gratitude verbally each day can result in increased alertness, enthusiasm, determination, attentiveness, energy, and quality of sleep, as well as the ability to sleep longer. A study done by Dr. Robert A. Emmons of the University of California and Dr. Michael E. McCullough of the University of Miami showed that those individuals who practiced weekly gratitude were more optimistic and felt better about their lives than were people who didn't practice weekly gratitude.

During the study, one group wrote about things they were grateful for what had occurred during the week. A second group wrote about daily irritations or things that had upset them. A third group wrote about events that had affected them but there was not

---

47   Linda Wasmer Andrews, "How Gratitude Helps You Sleep at Night," *Psychology Today* (blog), November 11, 2011, www.psychologytoday.com/blog/minding-the-body/201111/how-gratitude-helps-you-sleep-night.

an emphasis on being positive or negative. The first group who wrote about what they were grateful for also exercised more and had fewer visits to the doctor than did those who focused on daily irritations.[48]

ATTITUDE IS EVERYTHING

As much as some of us would like to be able to control every aspect of our lives, we can't! But what you can control is your attitude toward what does happen to you. We all experience and continue to experience trying times in our lives. The *what* in these situations is less important than the *how*.

How you react and move through these particular situations will determine their effect on your physical, mental, and emotional well-being. Up to 40 percent of our happiness comes from how you choose to approach your lives. Especially during trying times, we tend to focus on all of our problems. We then get in the habit of focusing our attention on all the negative things happening in our lives.

What would happen instead if you switched that focus to all of the good things that happen to you each and every day? What if you took time daily or weekly to reflect on things you are grateful for in your life?

DON'T WORRY, BE HAPPY

Gratitude is the forgotten factor in happiness research.

People who have a strong disposition toward gratitude have the capacity to be empathetic and to take the perspective of others. They are also rated as more generous and more helpful. Grateful individuals place less importance on material goods, are less likely to judge

---

48   Robert A. Emmons, 2003, "Counting Blessings Versus Burdens: An Experimental Investigation of Gratitude and Subjective Well-Being in Daily Life," *Journal of Personality and Social Psychology* 84(2): 377-389.

their own and others' success in terms of possessions, and are less envious of others.

 ## GRATEFUL INDIVIDUALS:

- report higher levels of positive emotions,

- have greater life satisfaction,

- experience greater vitality,

- are more optimistic,

- are healthier,

- build strong relationships,

- handle adversity better, and

- experience lower levels of depression and stress.

EXERCISE YOUR GRATITUDE MUSCLE

In a sense, gratitude is like a muscle and requires regular exercise to stay fit and functional. When writing in a gratitude journal, aim to find new things to be grateful for each day. Instead of constantly writing down that you are grateful for your family, look for more specific moments to be grateful for.

Gratitude comes in a lot of forms: important relationships, the ability to take charge of your health by changing the way you eat, things that happen to you, things you achieve, or things you have done. You can write down one to five things each day in a gratitude journal or make a list and keep it in a place you will see it several times a day.

There are a couple of great apps for your smart phone if that is easier. Gratitude Journal, Gratitude Diary, Gratitude Journal 365, and Day One are some of the popular ones.

It is important to be specific when acknowledging gratitude. For example, "*Today I am grateful that my husband made dinner so I could relax and take a hot bath.*" Gratitude journaling is so effective because over time it changes your perception of situations and what you focus on. Make it a point to notice new things each day to be grateful for. Here are several different ways to practice gratitude:

- Write a thank-you note.
- Thank someone mentally.
- Keep a gratitude journal.
- Meditate.
- Count your blessings.

Any time you set out to form a new habit, there will always be obstacles to face. You will quickly negate any benefits of practicing gratitude or journaling the things you are grateful for if you are beating yourself up about not being consistent with it. As with any change, set yourself up for success.

If you know that writing in a gratitude journal before bed isn't realistic for whatever reason, pick a different time of day. Or you may use a different form of expressing gratitude such as a gratitude jar. A gratitude jar is a jar where you place small pieces of paper with moments of gratitude written on them. You can review them weekly, monthly, or once a year.

We encourage you to start, continue, or resume a regular practice of expressing gratitude. Observe and notice the improvements in your mood, health, well-being, and overall happiness. Find a system that works for you and start small. Each day write down *one* gratitude statement and build from there.

chapter 25

MANAGING YOUR MINIMUMS

Janell learned about managing your minimums from a Precision Nutrition program. Minimums are the one to five behaviors that you have identified having the biggest impact on how you look, feel, and perform. Throughout your journey, you have noticed how certain things (food, behaviors, activities) make you feel physically, mentally, and emotionally. Now it's time to recognize what those things are and plan to consistently do more of the things that matter most.

Humans differ from one person to the next. It is important for you to tune into and recognize what works best for you and your body. Notice and name when you are feeling good, full of energy, and successful. This may not only require you to really pay attention, but it may also take some experimenting.

Questions to ask yourself as you identify your minimums:

- What habits or behaviors do you perform consistently?

- Which small changes that you have made have made a *really* big difference?

- What makes you feel good physically, emotionally, and mentally?

- What things make your body work best?

Be aware that at any given point your minimums may shift and change a bit. This could be due to a variety of things: your activity level, your stress level, or your health situation, to name a few. For example, when your activity level increases, you may need to focus on having the right types of carbs, in the right amounts, and at the right times.

Another way to think of your minimums is like a set of instructions for what you need—your own personal owner's manual.

 ## EXAMPLES OF MINIMUMS

- getting eight hours of quality sleep

- eating protein at each meal

- getting in eight thousand steps each day

- drinking half of your body weight in ounces of water per day

- avoiding gluten

- eating five to seven servings of non-starchy vegetables each day

- practicing self-care daily

Think foundational behaviors. Minimums are behaviors/habits (things you have control over), not outcomes.

Your minimums are ideally behaviors/habits that you are able to perform just about 100 percent of the time. When you are traveling or life gets in the way, you still pay attention to your minimums and make them happen. If not, it might be time to reevaluate and shift what your minimums are.

The purpose and idea behind managing your minimums is to give you a small number of behaviors/habits to focus on at one time. Pick the few things that make the greatest difference for you and focus your time and energy there. Then you can fill other things around your minimums.

INDIVIDUALIZE

Everyone is the same, yet everyone is different.

Human physiology is similar for all of us. For example, unlike cows, we all have one stomach and can't eat grass. However, you have probably discovered and learned a lot about yourself since you started this book. You know that what may work for your friend, family member, or coworker doesn't work quite the same for you. This is because we all have different stresses, environments, histories, and genetics. We all have our own unique stories; make this *your* journey, not someone else's.

For example, you may have noticed some foods make you feel better than others. Other foods don't make you feel good at all—you may have a food sensitivity that you didn't recognize before. You may feel better with cooked vegetables versus raw, or eating different types of carbohydrates. Some foods (or situations) may trigger certain behaviors that are not healthy.

Now that you have information about yourself and your body, it's time to individualize your nutrition to suit you even more. This doesn't mean making things more complex or difficult, often it means making things simpler. Decide exactly what you need as well as what fits into your life.

Making small, practical, and sustainable nutritional changes based on thoughtful, mindful, and informed self-awareness is the most sustainable way to make changes. Think about how you drive a car, you don't crank the steering wheel in one direction and then leave it there. You adjust as you drive along, whether you are driving in a straight line or making turns along the way.

The same principles apply with your supportive nutrition plan.

- Make small adjustments as necessary.

- Turn or backtrack when you need to.

- Work with *your* body's response and individual needs.

WHAT WORKS FOR YOU?

How do you know what works for you?

Ask yourself all or some of the following questions to figure out if what you are currently doing is working for you:

- Do you feel good inside and out?

- Do you have lots of energy for what you want to do?

- Are your health markers (blood chemistry, blood pressure, immune system, etc.) good?

- Are you meeting your goals?

Stay focused on consistently engaging in behaviors that give you the most return on investment in terms of your health and well-being.

chapter 26

PROGRESS, NOT PERFECTION

Some people give up due to slow progress, never grasping the fact that *slow progress is still progress.*

Many wrongly believe that a perfectionistic mind-set is motivating to achieve their goals when, in fact, it is anything but. This mind-set leaves you feeling "*not good enough*" much of the time. Why? Because most of the ideals we create in our mind are impossible to attain and are constantly changing.

We aren't talking about the worthy ideal we introduced in the mind-set section but instead things like the pictures we create in our head of an "*ideal body.*" That picture is always changing and, therefore, is always out of reach.

How does that motivate us to continue to making behavior changes and lasting transformation? It doesn't.

JANELL'S TIPS FOR GETTING PAST PERFECTIONISM

What Janell has discovered is that to be happy, stay positive, enjoy life, and actually achieve more, she must focus on where she is today versus where she used to be. For example, having the energy to train and move her body daily (where she is now) vs. lacking motivation and energy to work out and taking a nap every afternoon (where she used to be). From that perspective, things look much better! Try focusing on being better than you were, not on achieving perfection.

Stay consistent with your training schedule and focus on your progress, rather than an ideal created in your head. When you adopt a *Progress Not Perfection* mind-set, you can set new behavioral goals to work toward while still focusing on how far you have come and what you have accomplished. We all have progress and accomplishments that can be recognized! Look at the accomplishments you have made so far and use them as *fuel* for your progress forward.

PROGRESS NOT PERFECTION

The "progress not perfection" atmosphere at The Transformation Club has enabled me to continually better myself in so many areas of my life—not just working out. At the club, everyone works to his or her ability, and that feels so good. I know I can't lift the same weight as others, or I do wall sits instead of deep squats, but that's okay! I have increased the weights I can lift and I do a mean wall sit with weights. It is called progress. The progress in my workouts has given me confidence to improve my relationships and my eating habits, and even my sleep has improved. Not perfect but progressing!

—LuAnn Nead

HOW TO MEASURE CHANGE

Have you already experienced some level of transformation?

Today or sometime this week, set aside some time to reflect on *how you have changed?* Establish your current goals.

When asked this question about how you've changed, a few things may come to mind:

- the number on the scale

- how your clothes fit

- measurements

- progress photos

While the things included in the list can be tools to help you gauge change, we don't encourage or recommend *solely* using them to measure your progress. All of these measurement tools are based on outcomes versus behaviors. *Remember, we can control behavior goals but we can't control outcome goals.*

This is the very reason why we feel as though the scale is not the best measure of progress. Losing a certain amount of weight is an outcome goal. As much as you might think you can control outcomes, *you can't!* What you do have control over is the behaviors that lead you to a specific outcome. For example, eating six to eight servings of nonstarchy vegetables per day is a behavior that will help you to achieve a desired outcome of weight loss.

Ways to identify how you have changed:

- Are you focusing on doing what truly matters?

- Have you grown as an individual?

- Have you developed new life skills such as cooking or stress-management techniques?

- Do you now take control of your life and accept responsibility for your actions?

- Are you proactive; planning and strategizing how to handle certain situations?

- Has your emotional and mental health improved along with your physical health?

- Do you have more self-confidence?

- Do you ask for what you need?

- Do you eat foods regularly that you had previously not ever eaten or tasted?

- Have you overcome an obstacle or challenge that you once deemed impossible?

- Do you have more energy?

- Do you have a more positive outlook?

You may find these things harder to measure. Many of the things listed above are intangible but important. We believe they are *more important* than what the scale or measurements can tell you.

WHAT IS PROGRESS

If you are headed somewhere, how will you know when you get there? Oftentimes, if you are not paying attention, you will miss many signs along your journey. These are the things that tell you that you are moving in the right direction. They are the clear indicators that you are moving closer to your destination and making progress.

When you don't take time to identify and celebrate progress, you can miss it all together! We highly encourage you to stop, pause, and regularly look at how far you have come. It can be really motivating and exciting to see just how much you have changed physically, mentally, and emotionally.

What counts as progress for one person will be different from someone else. We are all at different places on our journey. Sometimes it can be hard to identify the progress in everyday life because you are seeing and living it every day.

Tangible progress is often easier to measure and see. Things such as your clothes fitting better, a decrease in weight, or improved health markers, like triglycerides. Those intangible things can be much harder to recognize.

Things like . . .
I feel confident in my food choices.
I am stronger inside and out.
I am better able to cope with stress.
I am happier.
I feel healthy.
I have become a better person.

When it comes to progress, track and identify what is important to *you*. This is your journey, not anyone else's. Looking at what you personally value and your goals is a good place to start. For many, a positive body image is important. Remember, don't hold onto unrealistic ideals. Instead of looking in a mirror and seeing the individual things you don't like, focus on what you do like and the progress you have made.

Keep an open mind about where you may find progress. As we have said before, the small things are sometimes the *big* things! *Anything* could be progress. Allow yourself to be a "work in progress."

STAYING POSITIVE

Even though you are focused on progress and not on perfection, there may be times where you find yourself reverting to old thought patterns. Just like everything else, it takes time to change old behaviors. When your mind has been working one way for many years, it isn't going to change overnight!

As humans, we are always measuring one thing to another. How and what we are measuring against can dictate our level of happiness. When we measure our achievements against an ideal that isn't attainable, we always feel as though we are *not good enough. Not doing enough.*

When you continue to use perfection as your guide for measurement, it can lead to low self-esteem, a state of unhappiness, and depression. Even though your achievements should make you accomplished, you are left very unhappy.

TIPS FOR HAVING A PROGRESS MIND-SET

You will likely have moments or days when you find yourself measuring your achievements against the idea of perfection or even measuring against others' progress/results. As we stated earlier, it will take some time and practice to shift your thinking. Following are some tips and tools to use when you find yourself feeling like you are coming up short as it relates to achieving your goals:

- **Write down your goals and review your progress weekly or daily.** If you don't have clearly defined goals, it can be hard to know when/if you are making progress. Focus on behavior goals versus outcome goals.

- **When you achieve a goal, acknowledge your success and then *celebrate*!** We are too quick to move on after an achievement. Give yourself the opportunity to take some time to celebrate.

- **Be present.** As a result of chasing perfection, life for some people is always spent thinking about the future. Practice appreciating the "here and now."

- **Practice gratitude.** Each day write down one to three things that you are grateful for. This does a couple of things: first it helps you to always look for the positive in every situation, and second, it will help you to acknowledge achievements.

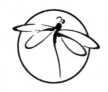

chapter 27

LIFE BEYOND THIS BOOK

This book is quickly coming to an end. You may have mixed feelings about this. Maybe you aren't ready to apply the principles we have covered. Maybe you don't feel confident that you can do this on your own. Maybe you are afraid of failure. Maybe you are excited about all the knowledge you have gained.

All of this is okay. Know that most of the time no one is 100 percent ready for anything. Trust that you can handle whatever life brings you. It is likely that you will fail; if/when you do, *get back up*! When we experience a failure or setback, we use it as information moving forward. There are no such things as failures, only opportunities to learn. Remember that you can always refer back to the content in this book.

We want to leave you with several points to help you to continue to move forward with your journey.

CREATING AND MAINTAINING
HEALTH IS A LIFELONG EVENT

Here are some thoughts to keep in mind as you pursue health for the long term:

- **Go back to foundational behaviors first.** You can always go back to the basics. These are the things that are at the core of your supportive nutrition plan and healthy lifestyle: protein, nonstarchy vegetables, healthy fats, appropriate amounts of carbohydrates, sleep, and stress management.

- **Be your own coach.** Constantly ask yourself, *How is this working for me?* If it's not, then change something. Do this with honesty and self-compassion.

- **Take action.** Ask yourself, *What can I do today to move me forward in a positive way?* Keep it simple and then do that.

- **Ask for help when you need it.** Build a solid support system. Surround yourself with like-minded people. Don't try to be a hero; if you need help, ask for it. Stay connected to individuals and communities of people who will move you forward.

- **Working on the inside is just as important as the outside.** Being healthy goes far beyond grams of carbohydrates, meal planning, and grocery shopping. It all begins with who you are on the inside. You don't have a good chance of staying healthy and achieving your goals without the support and help of your mind, heart, and soul.

- **Trust the process.** Behavior changes that last a lifetime are often slow. Your progress may also be slow. Practice patience.

When you engage in healthy behaviors consistently, results will follow.

- **Know what foods work for you and which work against you.** From the content in this book, you know what foods will nourish your body and support your goals. Begin to identify which foods are "trigger" foods for you and that you tend to overeat. Embrace the foods that truly support you physically, mentally, and emotionally, and don't be fooled by those that don't.

- **Your body knows best.** Listen to the signals your body gives you and trust that it knows what it is doing. Help it by eating slowly. Let it be your guide as to when you are hungry and when you are full.

- **Eat for nourishment.** Eat to nourish your body physically, mentally, and emotionally. Your body is a truly amazing organism that does so much for you. Reward it by providing it with proper nutrition from whole, real, unprocessed foods. Food should also taste good and be satisfying. Don't deprive yourself and rely on fake convenient "diet foods." If you want something like a dessert, cookie, muffin, or pancake, then make it the highest quality possible.

- **Allow yourself and your priorities to evolve.** Things will inevitably change when it comes to your nutrition and healthy lifestyle. Your priorities may shift from fitting into a pair of jeans to gardening or buying local meat and produce. Remember that just because something worked for you in the past doesn't mean it will always work. Our bodies are shifting and changing just like our lives. Your body may need something different than it once did.

- **Prioritize self-care.** If you don't prioritize yourself, your self will suffer. Self-care is not selfish. It's essential to our health and well-being.

- **Progress is anything that you define as progress.** If progress to you is eating one piece of pie at your next holiday gathering instead of three, then that's progress. You define what progress and success means to you. Then establish which behaviors will move you toward that. Engage in those behaviors consistently, and then celebrate your progress and success.

- **Manage your minimums.** Decide what behaviors you will do 95–100 percent of the time and then do them without fail. Set your guidelines and then when "life happens," just focus on your minimums and let that be good enough for now.

- **Give back.** Help someone else with their nutrition and lifestyle choices. Share your experience.

Creating a supportive nutrition plan and leading a healthy lifestyle is a lifelong event.

Congratulations for taking another step in the direction of creating and leading a healthier lifestyle. Acknowledge that you purchased this book and read the content on how to become a better version of yourself. That takes time, effort, and courage! We applaud each and every one of you!

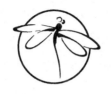

afterword

IT'S *NOT* ABOUT THE WEIGHT LOSS

We've helped literally thousands of people lose weight and get in great shape. Our hope is that this book will dramatically multiply the number of lives we transform. B*ut*, and this is a *big but*, for us, **it's not about the weight loss.**

It's about the life-changing stories we get to be a part of.

It's the tired, burnt-out mom who lost herself years ago that now has self-confidence and a new purpose and is the example for her children she always wanted to be.

It's the young woman who struggled her whole life with body image issues who became healthy, strong, and proud of who she is and what she can offer to the world.

It's the busy dad who got so wrapped up in his career that he was missing out on his family, all the while slowly killing himself with caffeine and sugar to keep up and alcohol and late-night TV to wind down. Now he's a true leader for his family, putting his health at the top of the priority list so he can truly be the best provider possible.

It's the couple who hasn't been connected in years, just going through the motions wondering when things will be different. Now they enjoy cooking healthy meals together and see their workouts as daily dates.

We've been fortunate enough to see so many of these truly life-changing stories—real-life *transformations*.

That is what it's all about.

That is what we want for you.

That is what drives us each and every day.

Our mission is to educate, motivate, and inspire you to become the BEST version of YOU.

We wholeheartedly believe (and we've got tons of empirical evidence to prove it) that when you take the best care of yourself following the guidelines we've shared with you in this book, then you will not only transform your life to be happier, healthier, and more fit, you will transform the lives of everyone around you.

That may sound a bit extreme, but it's true. We understand that it's hard for some people to believe that "little ol' me can impact the world," but you do. At the smallest end of the spectrum, your happiness *will* brighten the day of those around you. We see that all the time when our members come into The Transformation Club after a tough day at work. Their whole mind-set shifts when they walk in and see the smiling faces and positive attitudes of our team and their fellow workout partners. Members also tell us how their coworkers have said they do the same for them when they come into work now. Your happiness might improve a coworker's performance that day or translate into a better family dinner experience for her that night.

On the other end of the spectrum, you *will* inspire someone to make their own transformation—changing their life dramatically, and as such, the lives of those around them. We see this all the time also. In fact, referrals are a big part of how we've built our business. It simply starts with one person transforming his or her life and then inspiring one more person to do the same.

Who will you inspire? Whose life will you transform?

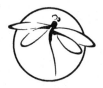

how to get started

The best way to protect yourself from putting your transformation off is to set a deadline and *start now*.

Deadlines are powerful motivators. Without a deadline, you really have no endpoint toward which to work. You have nothing to push you when obstacles present themselves—they always do!

Without a deadline, tomorrow never comes.

IT'S TIME TO SHAKE THINGS UP

If you keep doing what you have always done, then you will get the results you have always gotten. It's time to do something different. Ask yourself this question:

"If I keep doing what I am doing right now, will I achieve what I want to achieve?"

If you answered no, then it's time for a change.

Get your calendar out and decide when you want to see your first wave of results. Be realistic: make sure you give yourself time to really dig in and see changes, but challenge yourself, too. Make it a little tough so you can take full advantage of the power of urgency.

Sometimes, a deadline may not be enough because you may be tempted to move it. Deadlines are not supposed to be moving targets! The best way to prevent deadline-creep is to get competitive. Entering into a competition, contest, or challenge is a sure way to give you the edge you need to keep yourself on track and finish strong. There is something very motivating about competing with others (or yourself). Just knowing that your effort and results are going to be measured alongside others really will give you an extra boost in motivation.

This is a time when a little peer pressure is useful! And you will find that those with whom you are in competition with will also be your biggest cheerleaders—they know exactly what you are going through and will be there to encourage you to keep moving.

START FAST AND FINISH STRONG!

Deadlines and contests are great ways to get you started and keep you on track to achieve your goals—put them to work for you now! To find out when our next Transformation Challenge begins, visit www. TheTransformationClub.fitness. We'd love to have you join us!

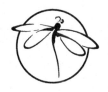

resources

The 7 Key Questions Every Personal Trainer You Hire Must Be Able to Answer

Visit **www.7QuestionsReport.com** to download this special report to learn the questions you need to ask and the answers you should receive when interviewing a personal trainer.

Janell's Top Ten Favorite Paleo Recipes

Visit **www.Top10PaleoRecipesBook.com** to download these easy-to-make Paleo-friendly recipes that you and your whole family will love.

21-Day Detox Challenge

The 21-Day Detox Challenge is a comprehensive program based around eating whole foods and eliminating common inflammatory foods. It is designed to help you identify how certain foods are affecting you physically, mentally, and emotionally. Through education, grocery shopping lists, recipes, and daily emails, you are set up for twenty-one days of success. Common results of this program include but are not limited to: more energy, sleeping better, weight loss, less joint pain, and clearer skin. For more info or to sign up, visit **www.21daydetoxchallenge.info**.

Books to Understand and Improve Your Mindset

As a Man Thinketh by James Allen or *As a Woman Thinketh* by James Allen & Justin Yule

The Power of the Subconscious Mind by Dr. Joseph Murphy

Psycho-Cybernetics by Maxwell Maltz

You Were Born Rich by Bob Proctor

Think & Grow Rich by Napoleon Hill

contact us

Website:

www.TheTransformationClub.fitness

Facebook:

https://www.facebook.com/
thetransformationclubchanhassen

Free Tips & Strategies to Lose Weight & Feel Great:

https://www.facebook.com/groups/
FREELoseWeightFeelGreat

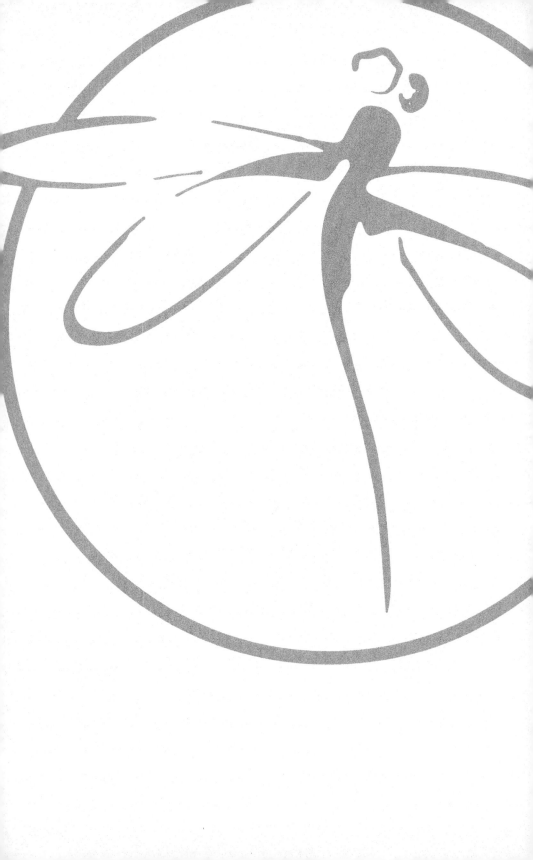